MY PICTURE BOOK OF

butterflies

Take your time, smile, and let these 80 beautiful butterflies brighten your day.

SILVER DOVE
BOOKS

Monarch

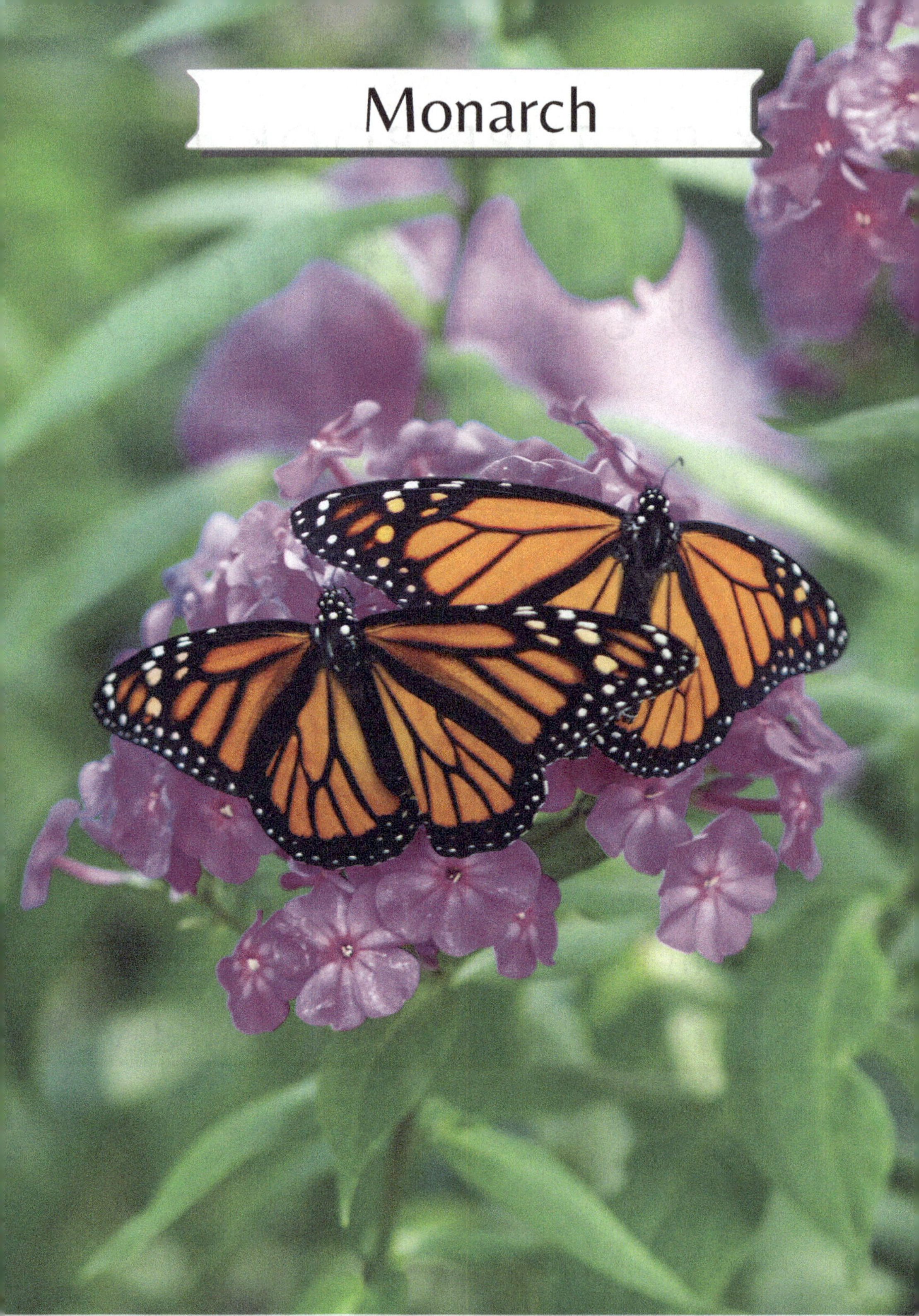

Monarchs migrate thousands of miles every year.

Cairns Birdwing

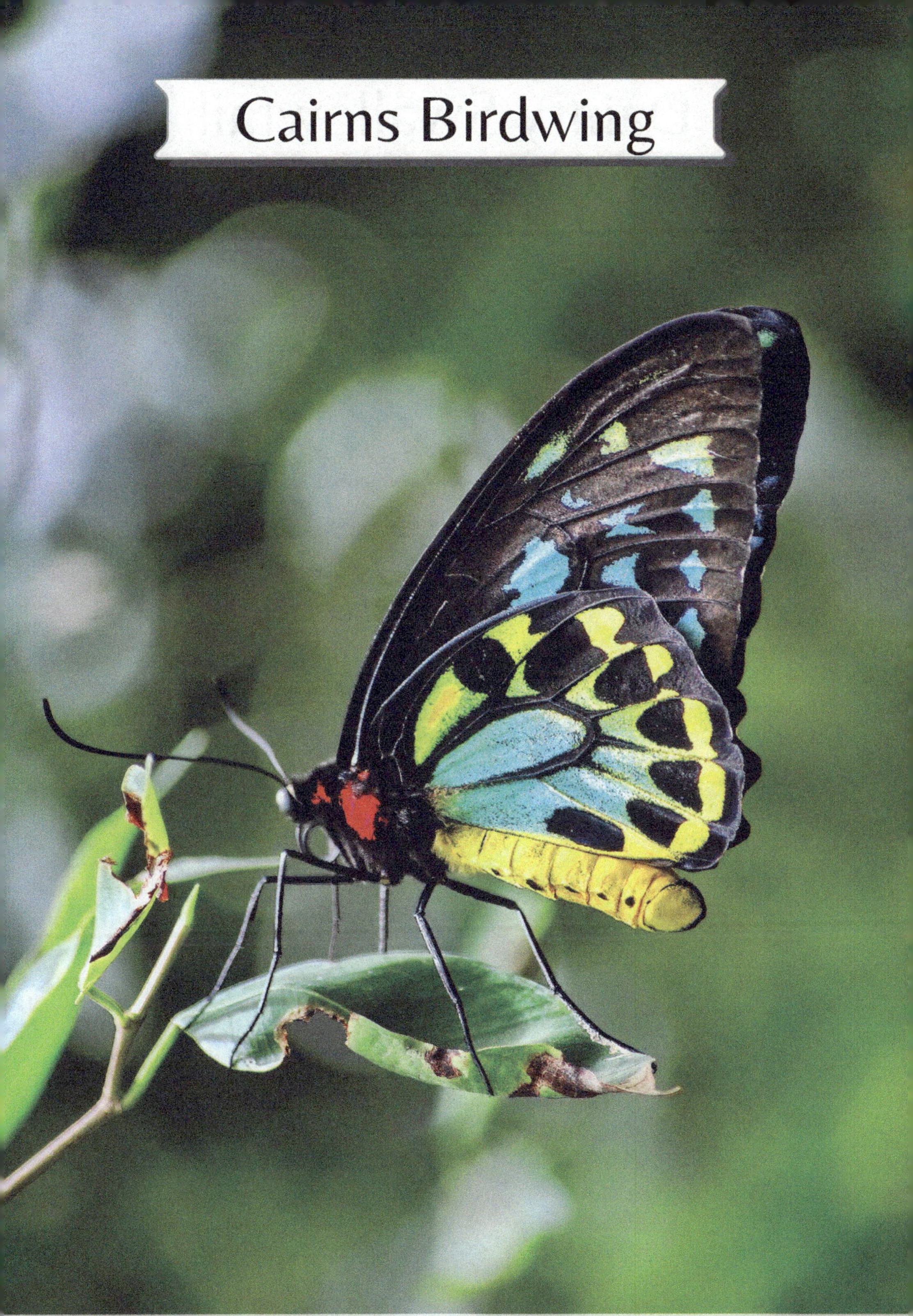

Australia's largest native butterfly.

Dainty Swallowtail

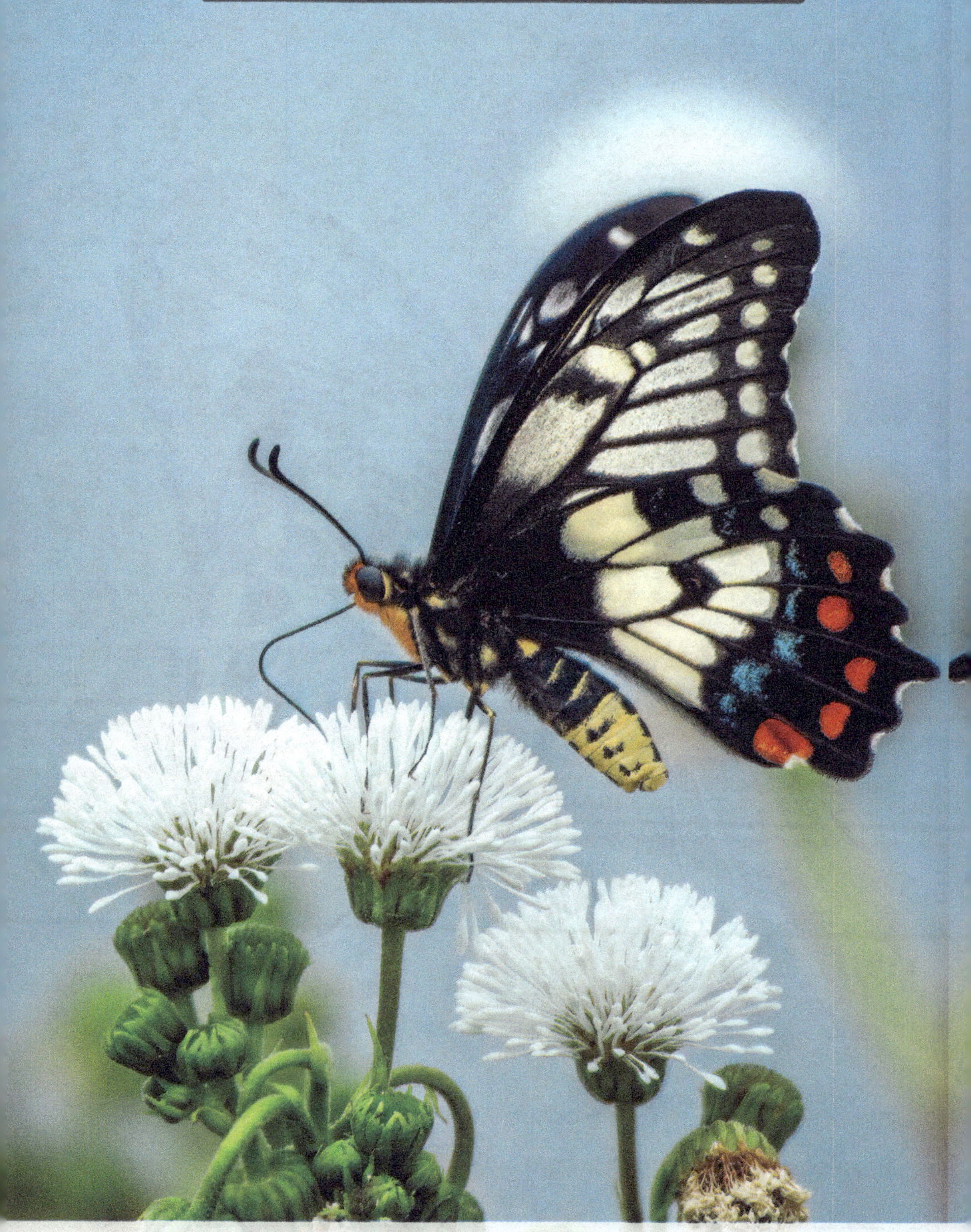

Feeds on citrus; found in Eastern Australia.

Purple Monarch

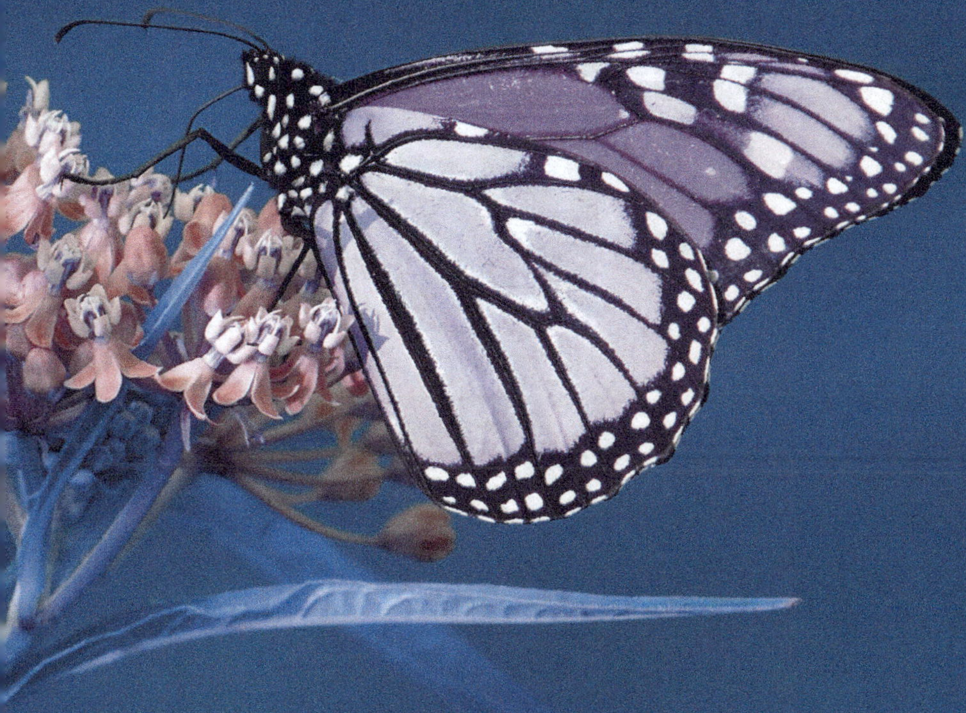

A rare, violet variant of the common monarch.

Blue Tiger

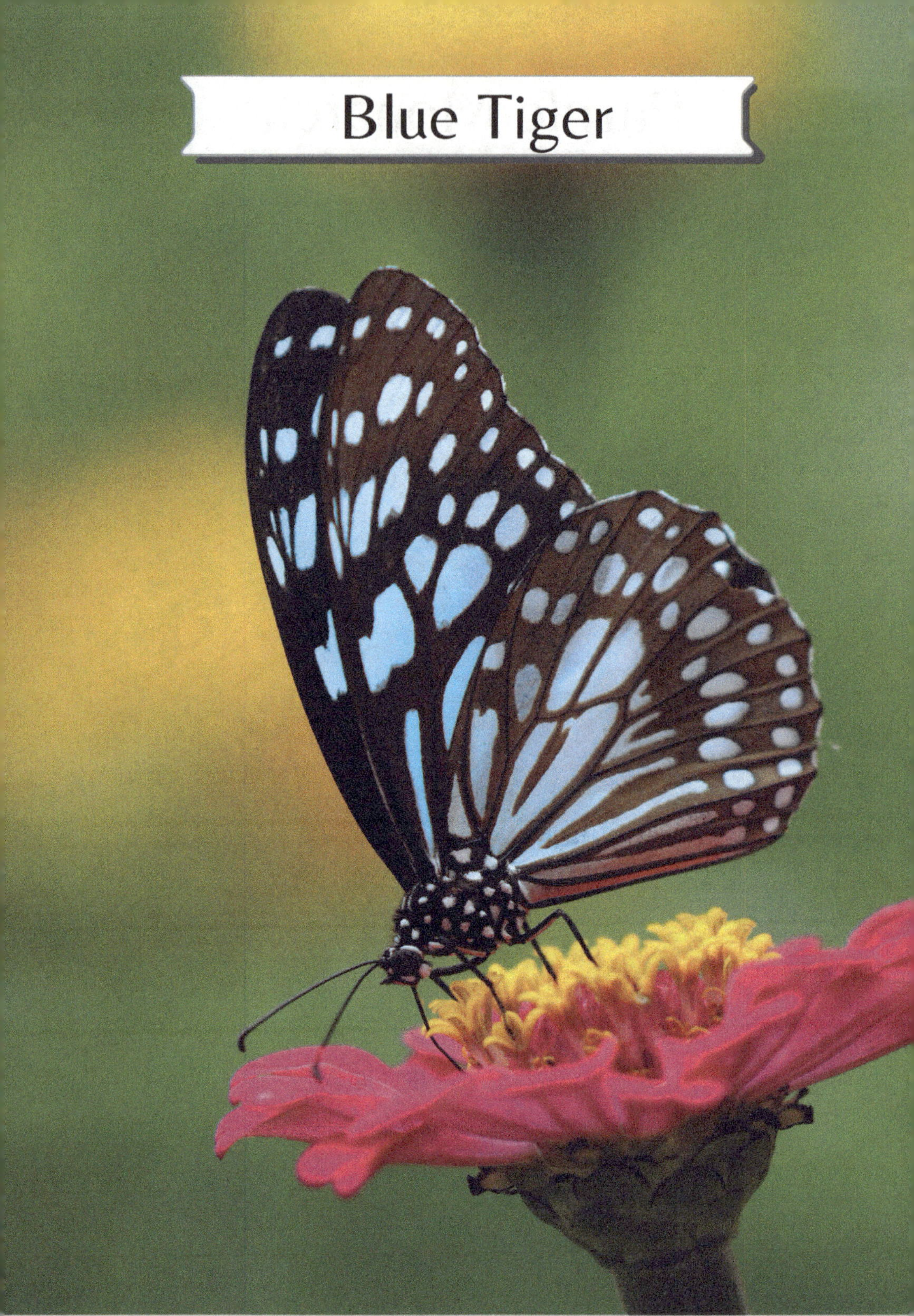

The blue and black stripes mimic toxic butterflies.

Adonis Blue

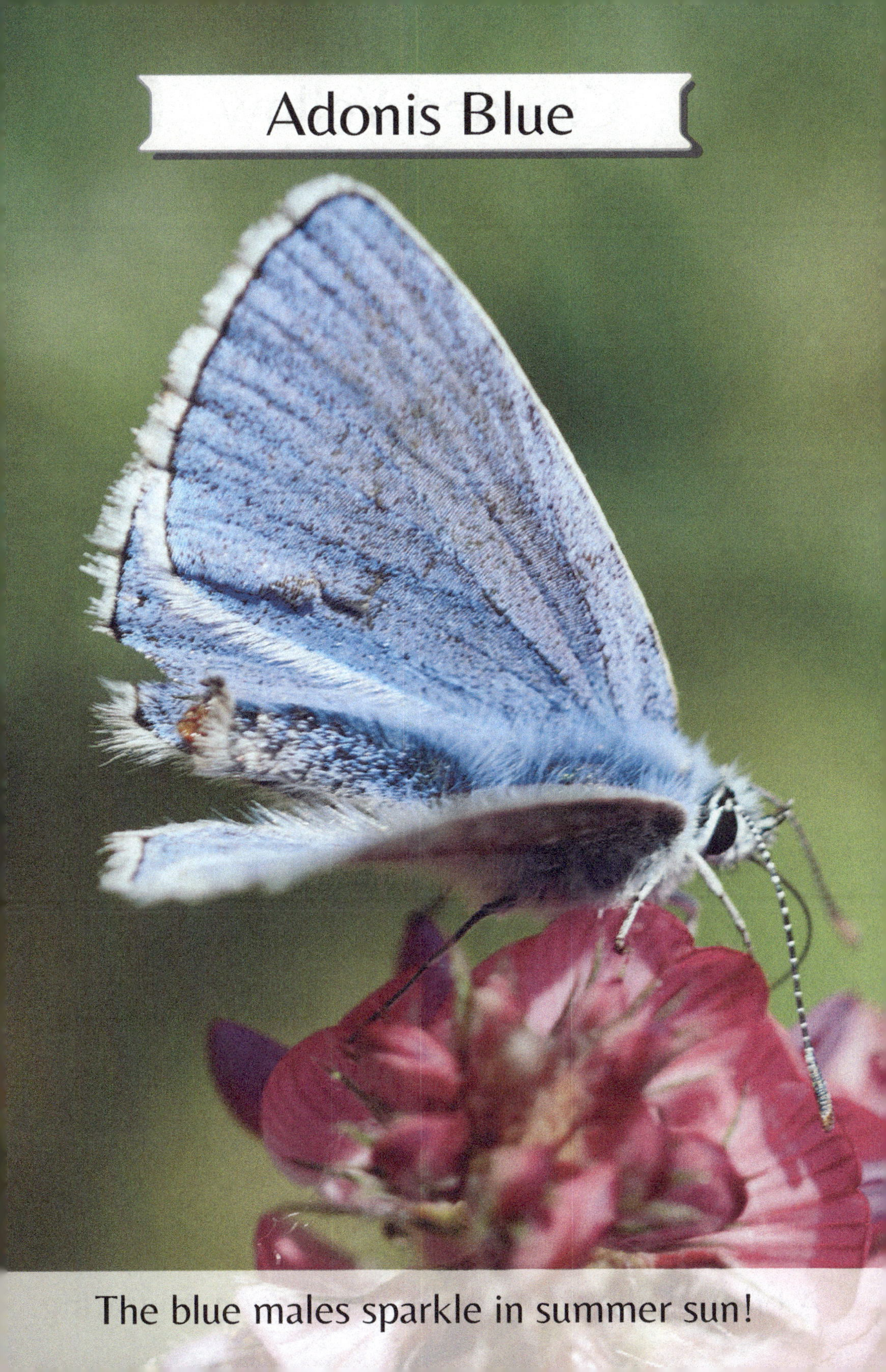

The blue males sparkle in summer sun!

Clouded Yellow

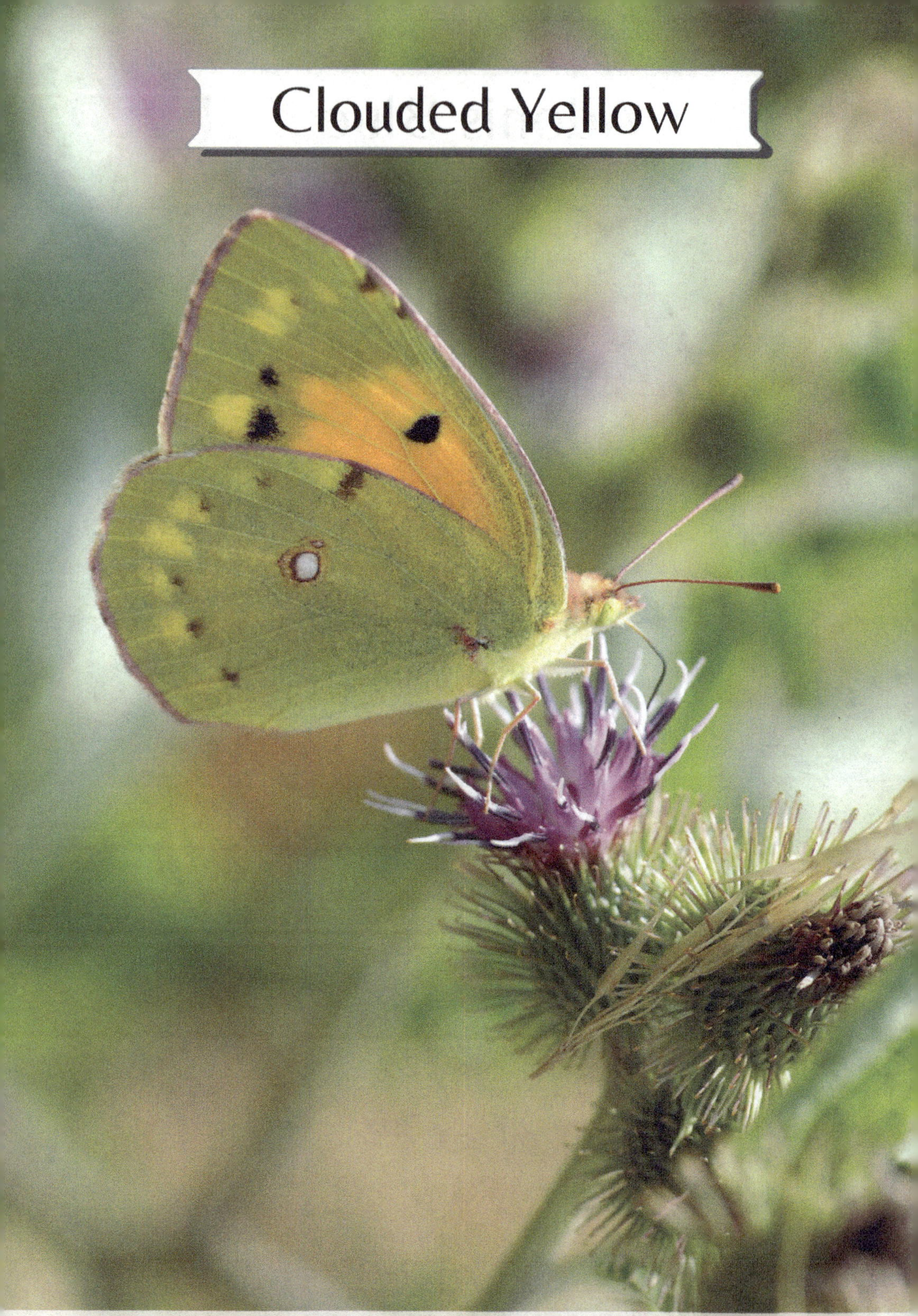

A bright yellow butterfly, often seen migrating.

Comma

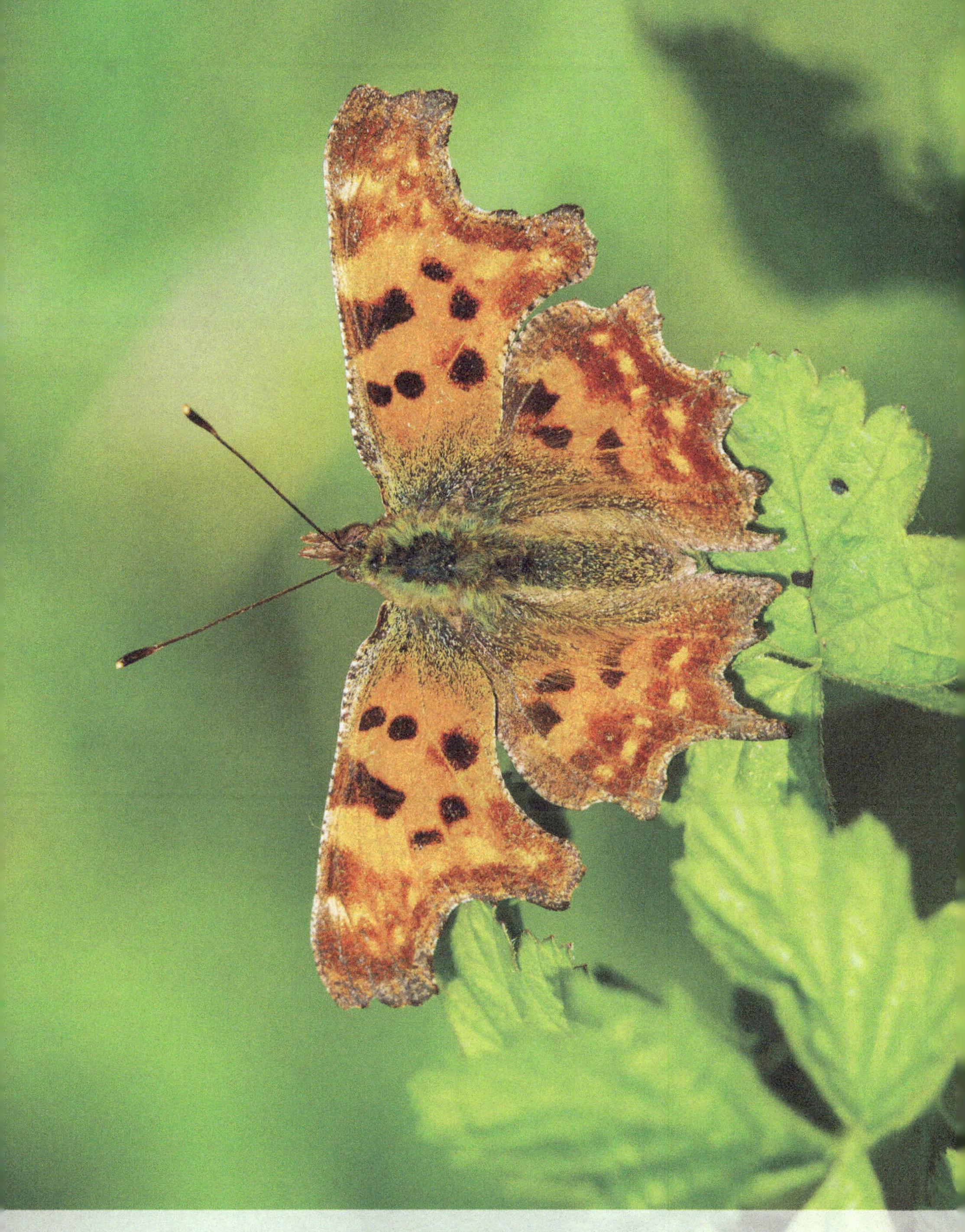

Has a comma-shaped mark underneath!

Common Blue

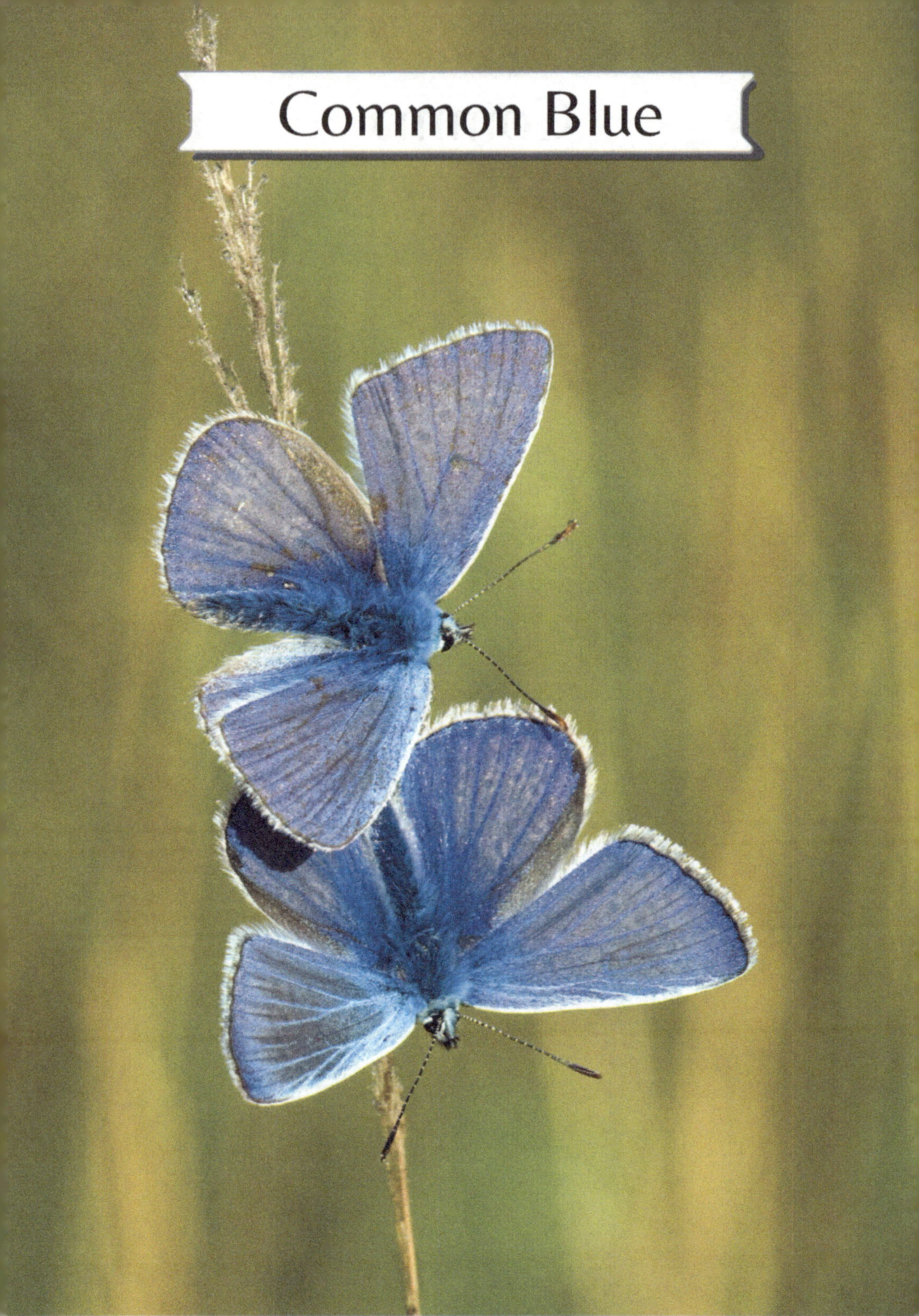

Widespread across Europe and loves wildflowers.

Dark Green Fritillary

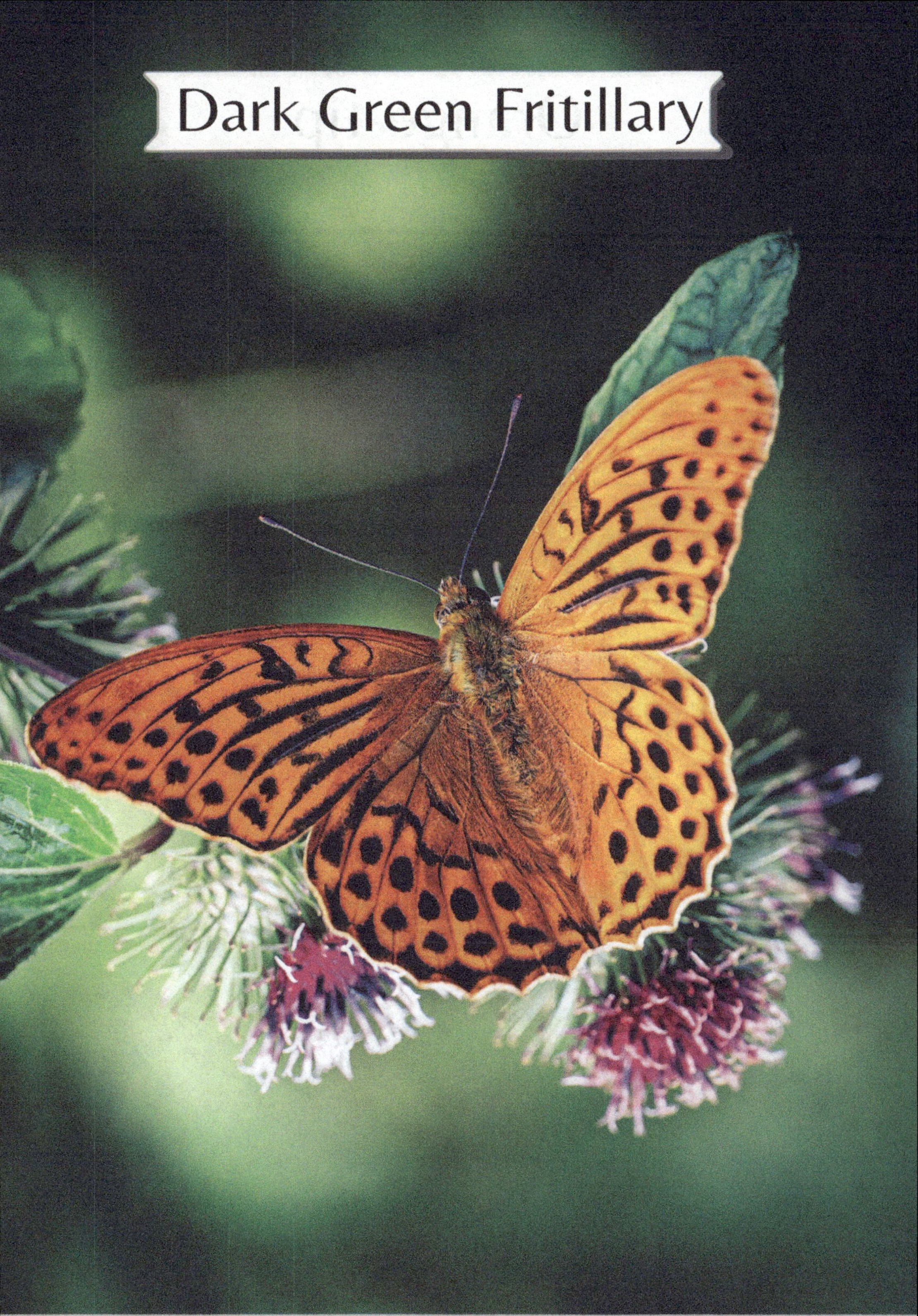

A fast flyer with greenish underwings.

Orange-tip

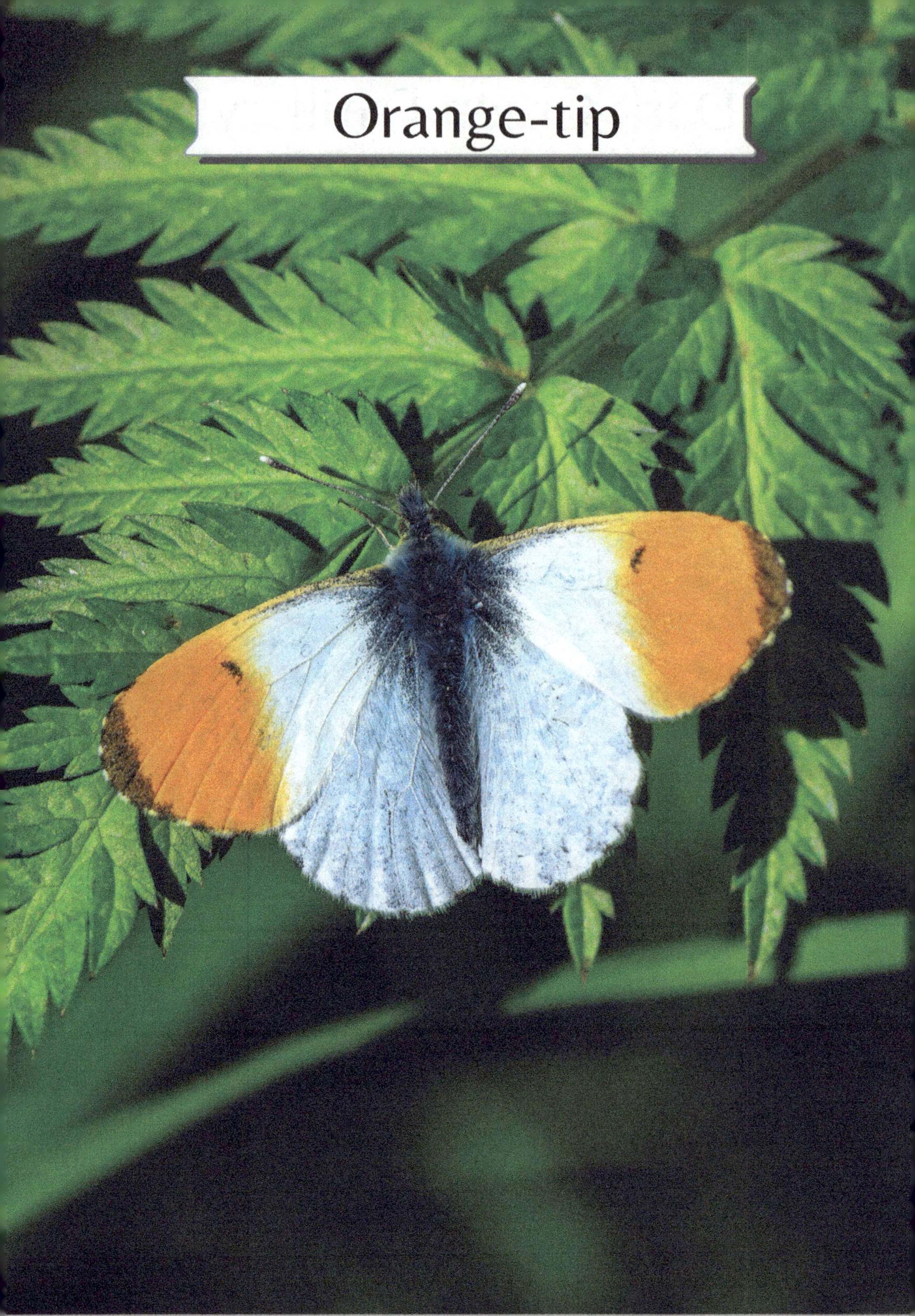

Only the males have bright orange wing tips.

Dingy Skipper

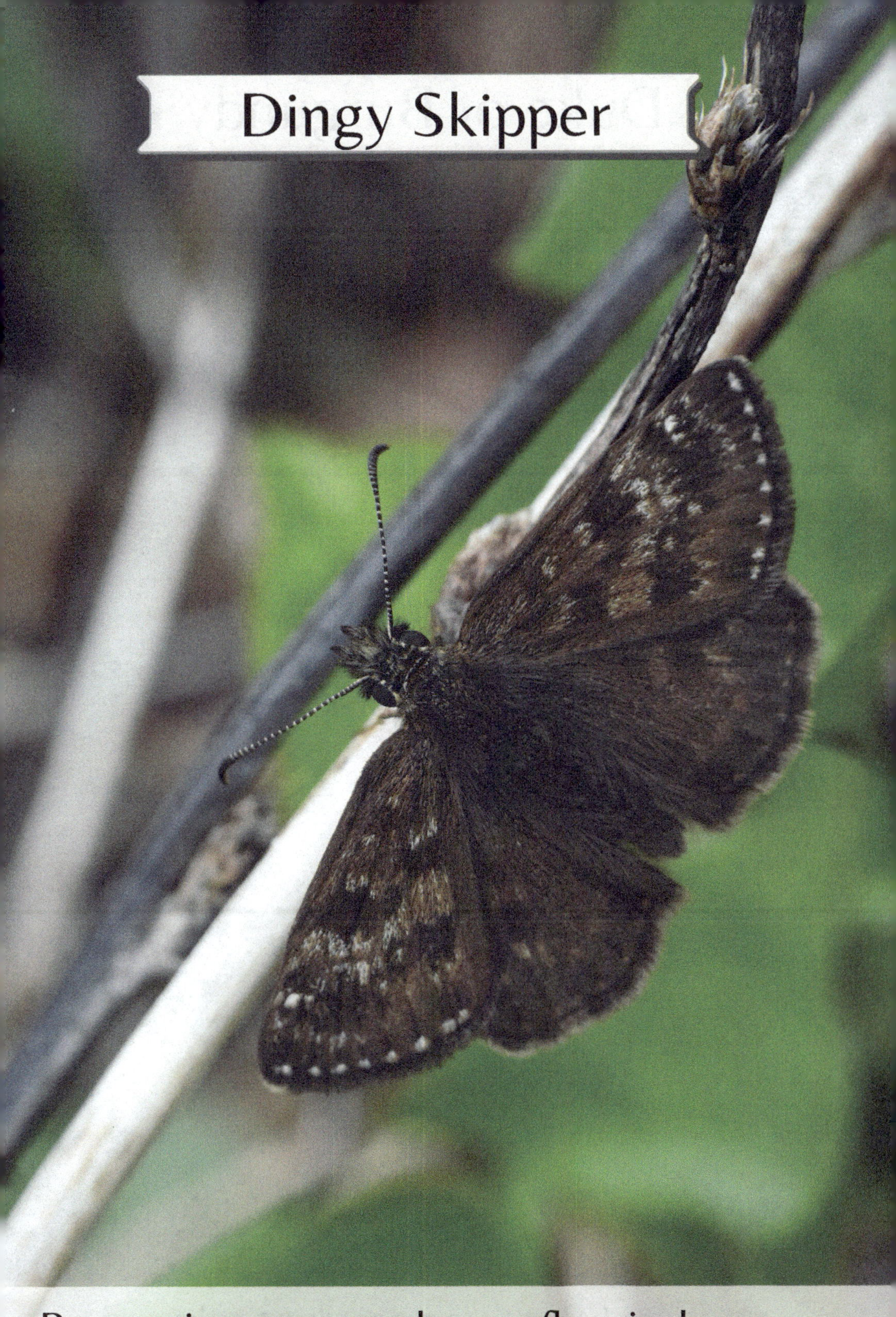

Brown wings are a good camouflage in dry grass.

Duke of Burgundy

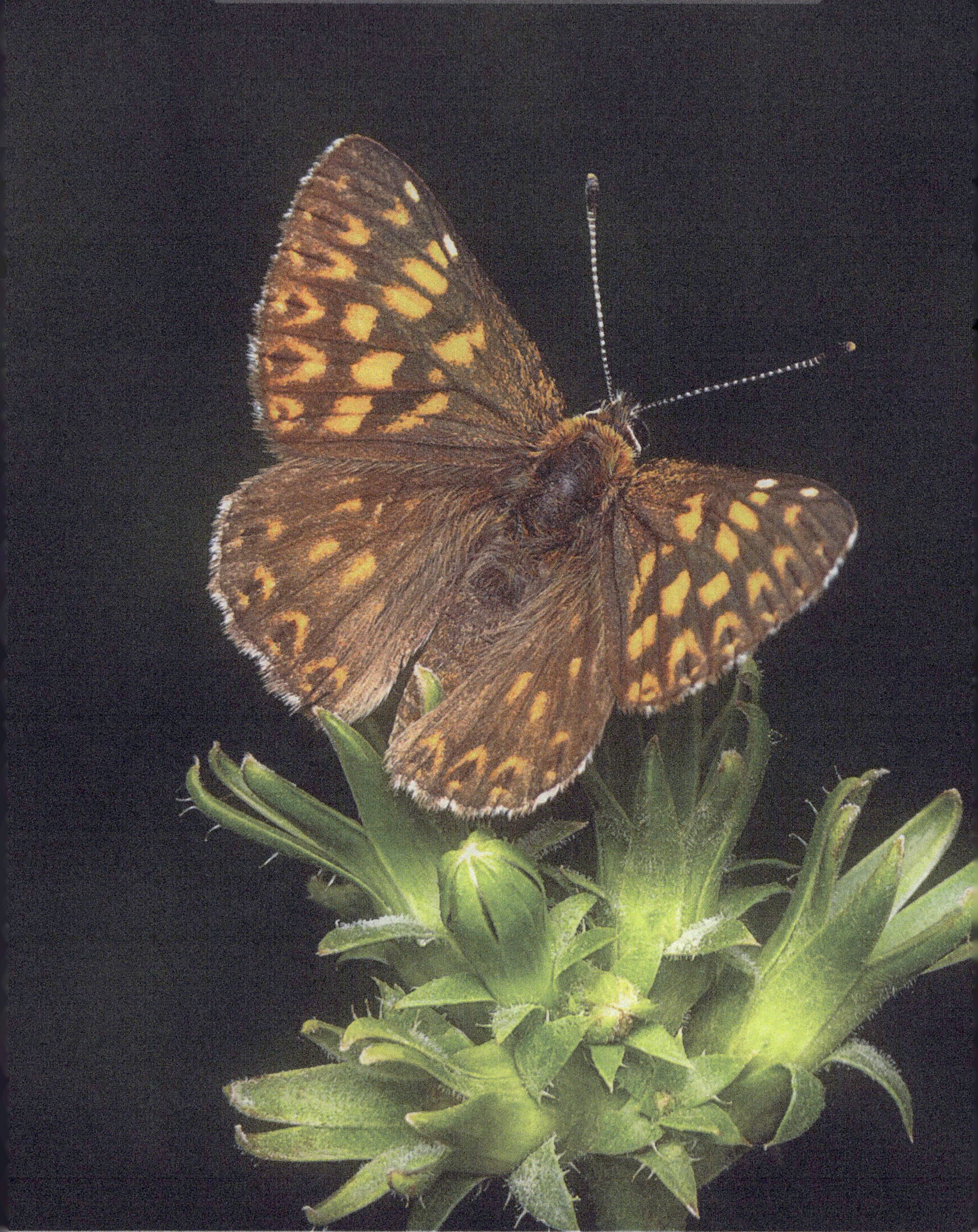

One of Britain's rarest butterflies.

Gatekeeper

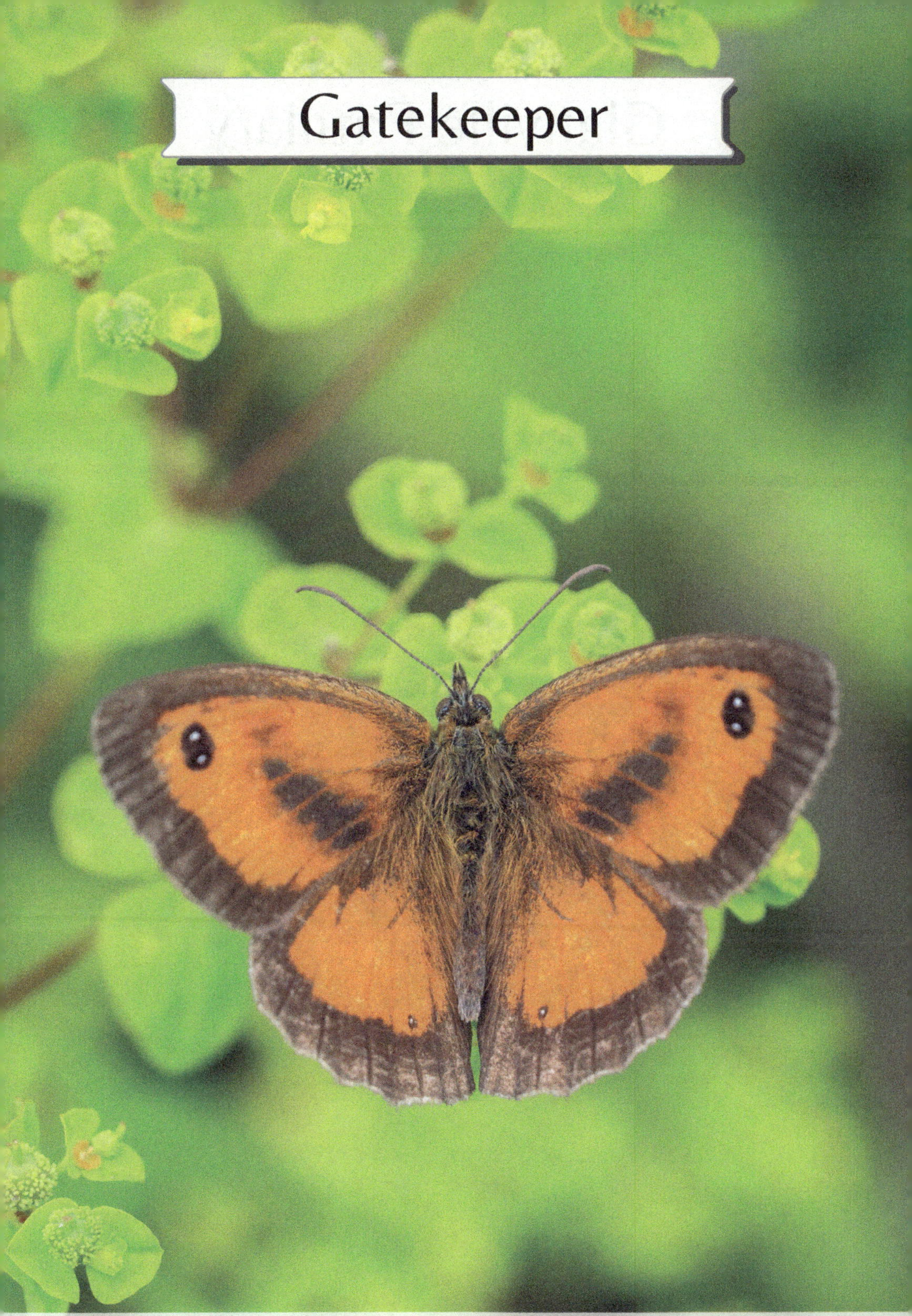

Gatekeepers are often seen near meadows.

Glanville Fritillary

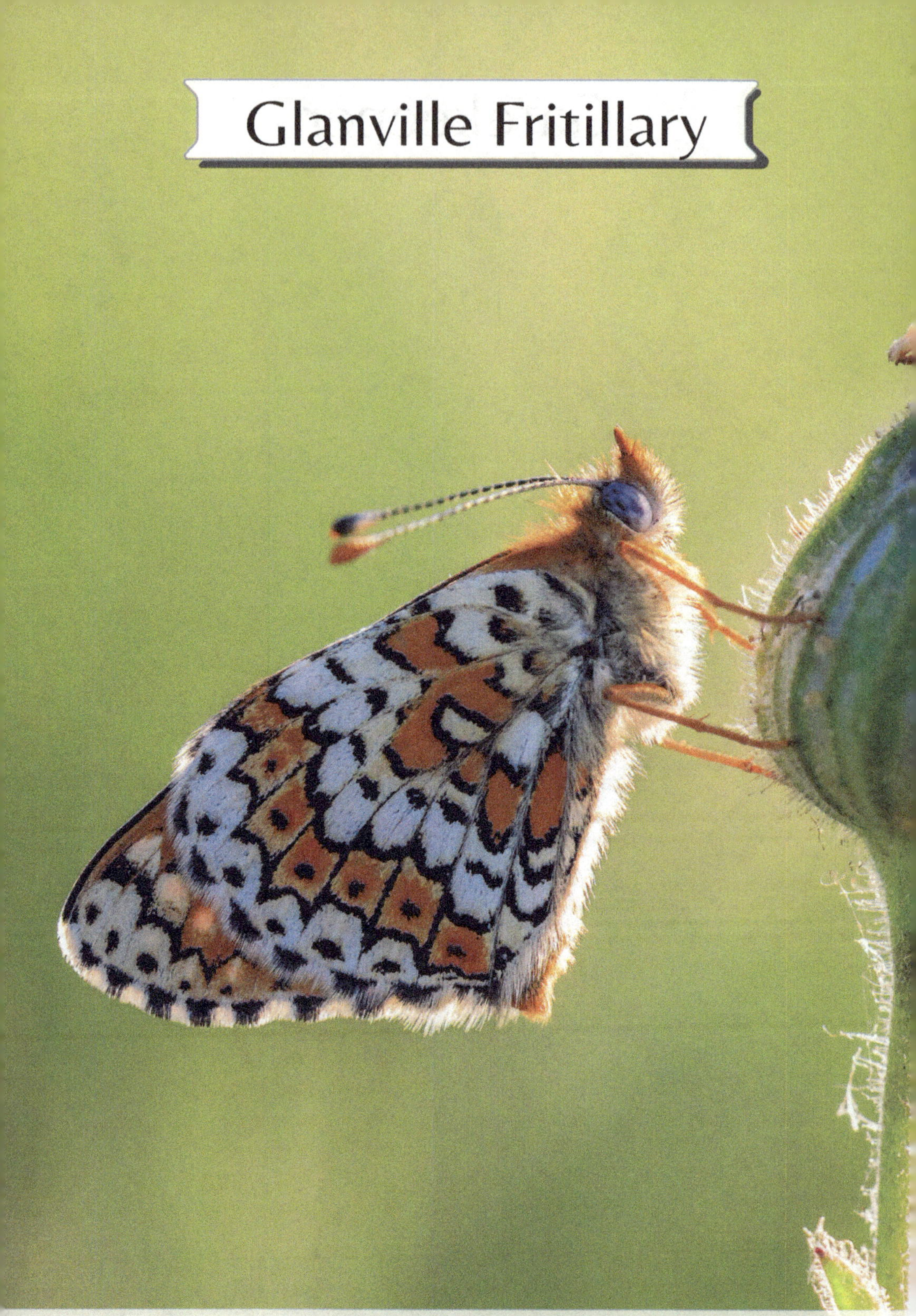

Found on coastal cliffs and meadows.

Grayling

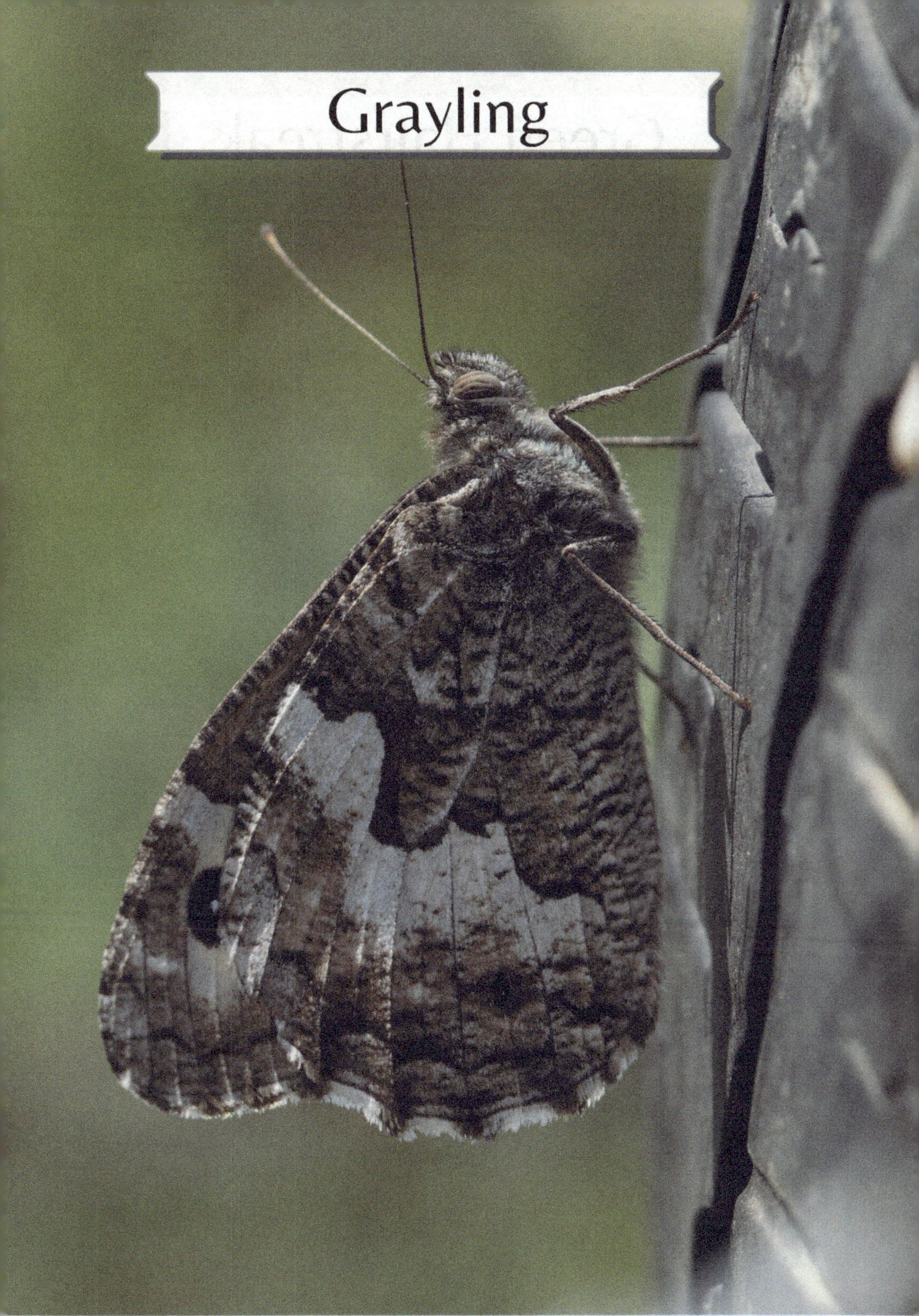

A master of camouflage on sandy and rocky ground.

Green Hairstreak

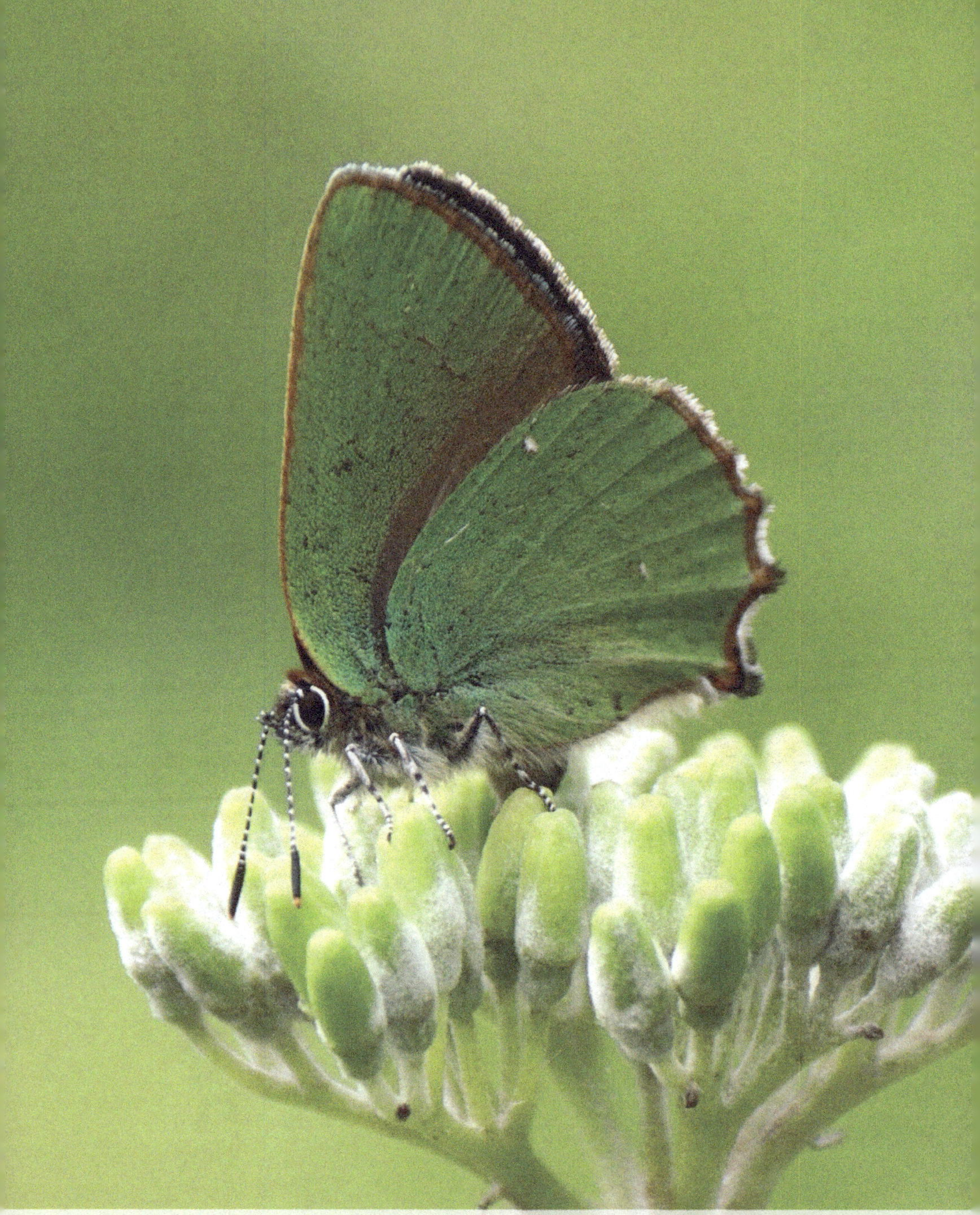

The only truly green butterfly in the UK.

Green-veined White

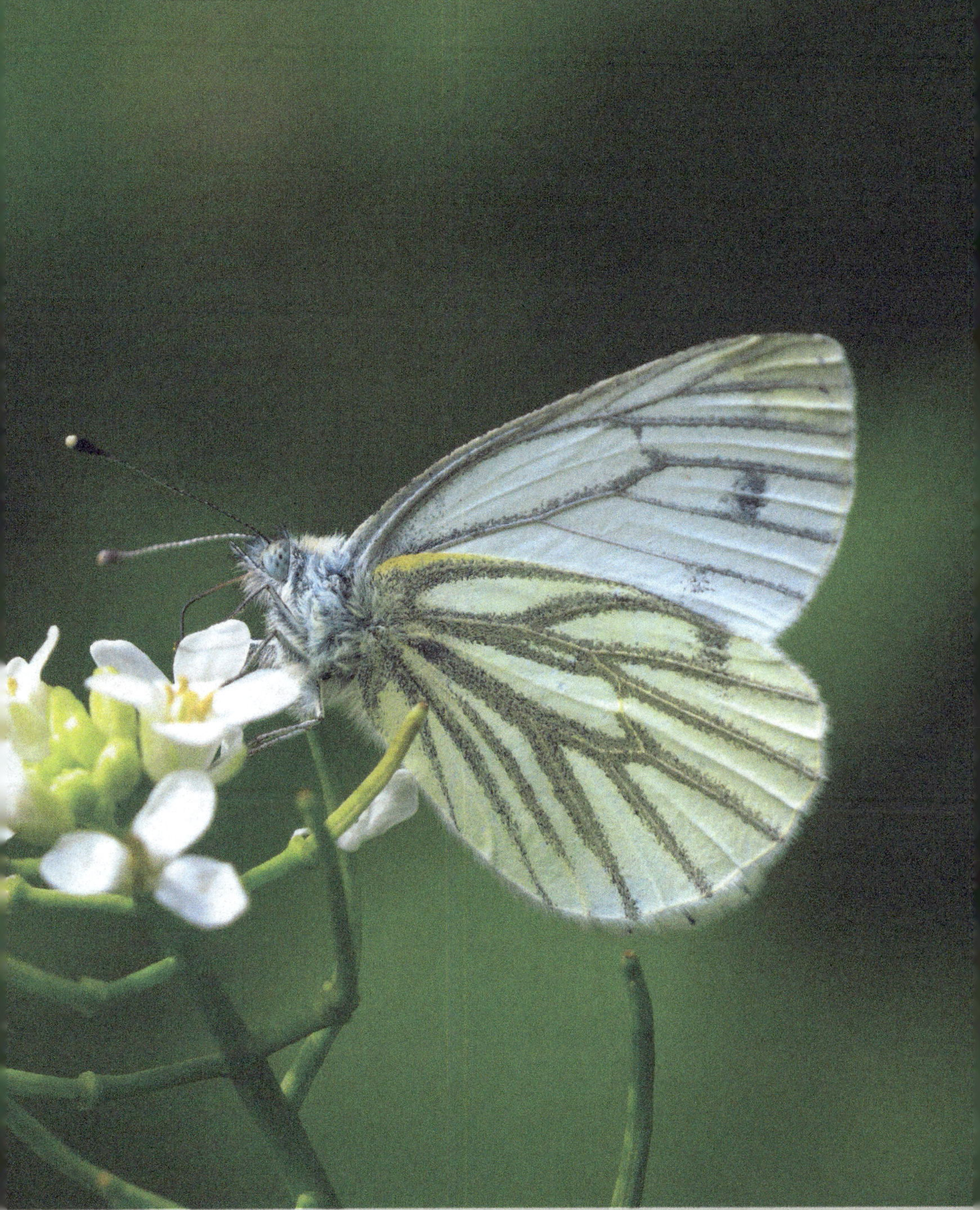

The green veins distinguish them from cabbage whites.

Grizzled Skipper

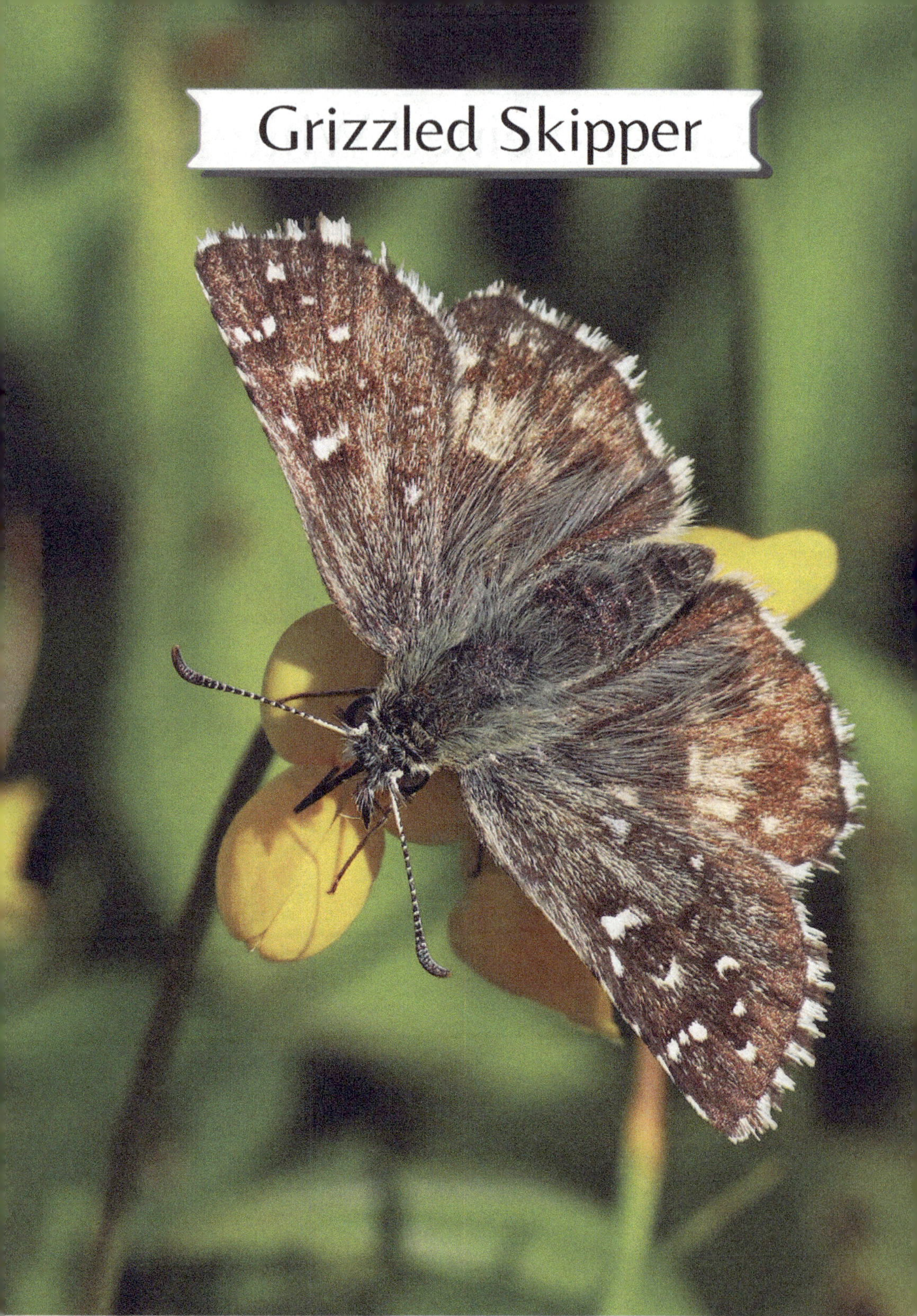

This small, checkered butterfly loves sunny patches.

Heath Fritillary

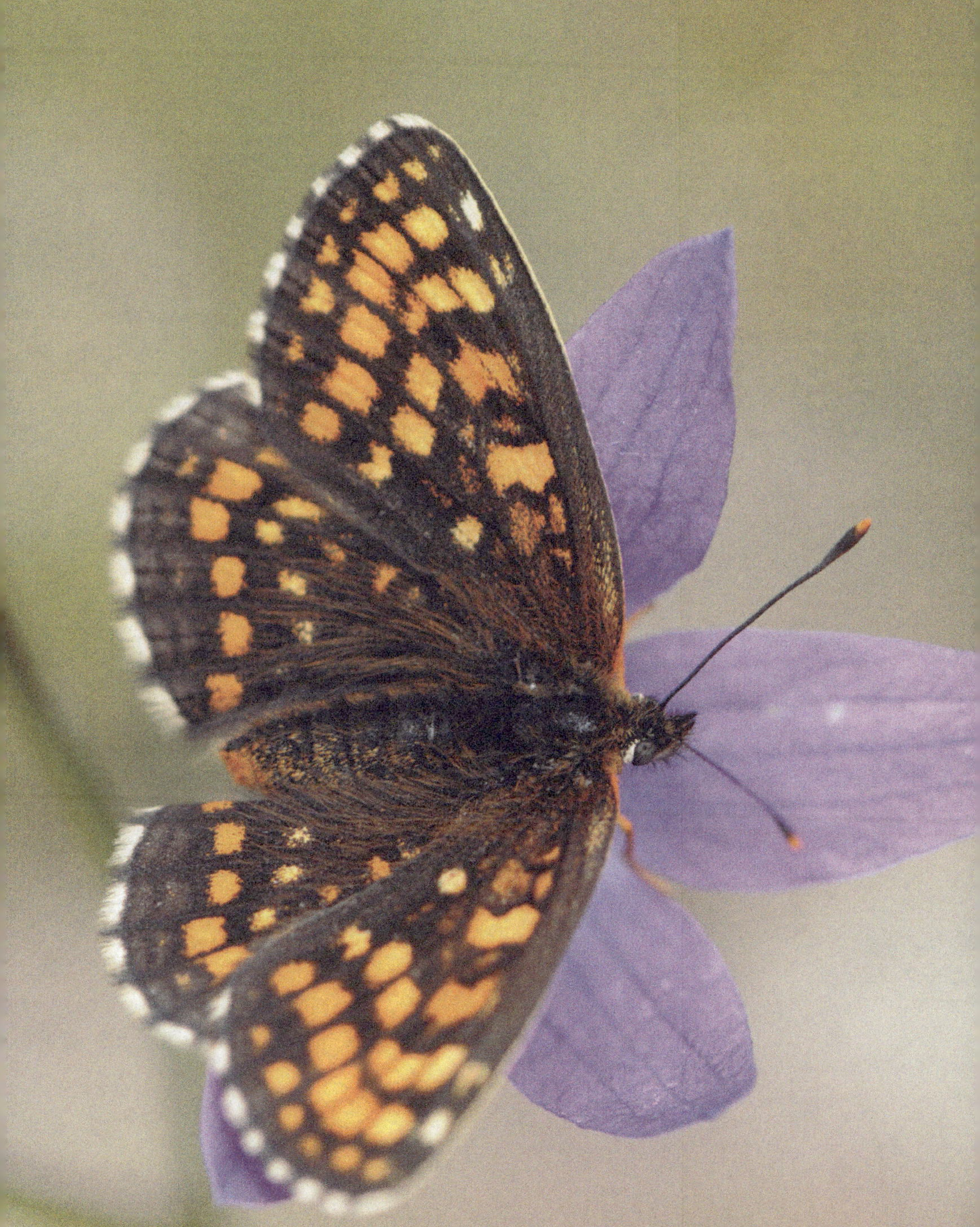

Found in sunny clearings and heathland.

High Brown Fritillary

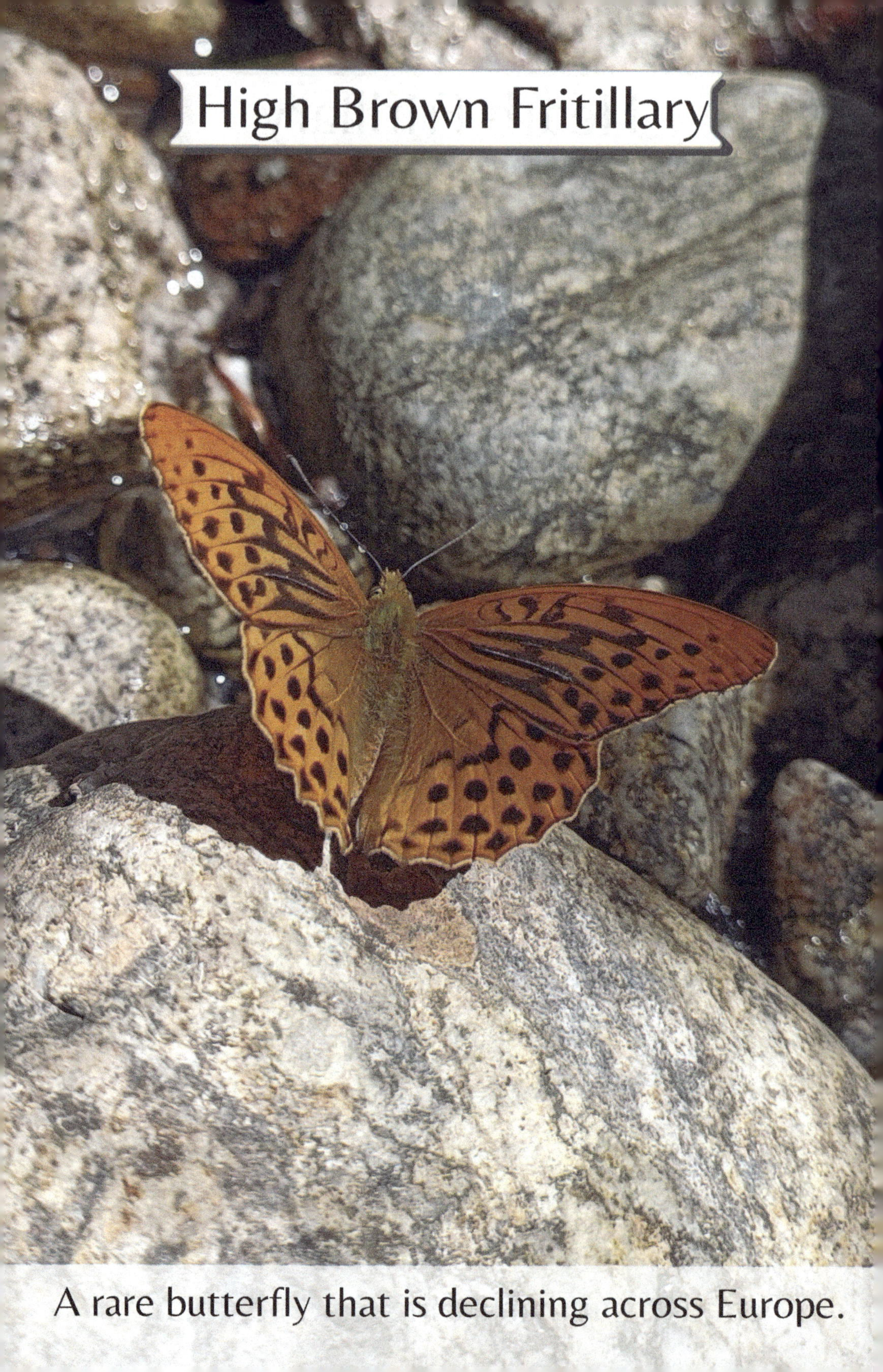

A rare butterfly that is declining across Europe.

Holy Blue

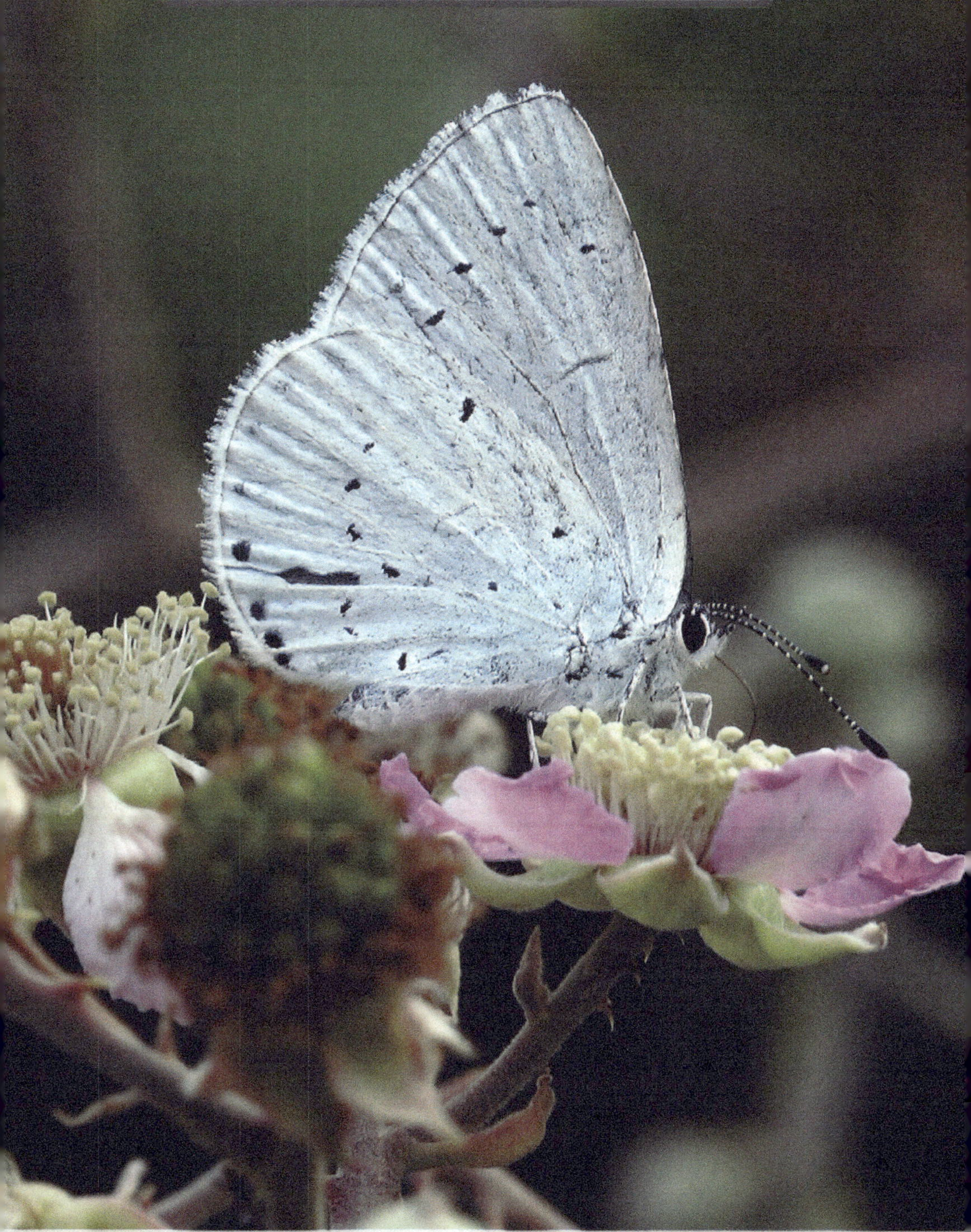

Found near holly and ivy plants.

Speckled Wood

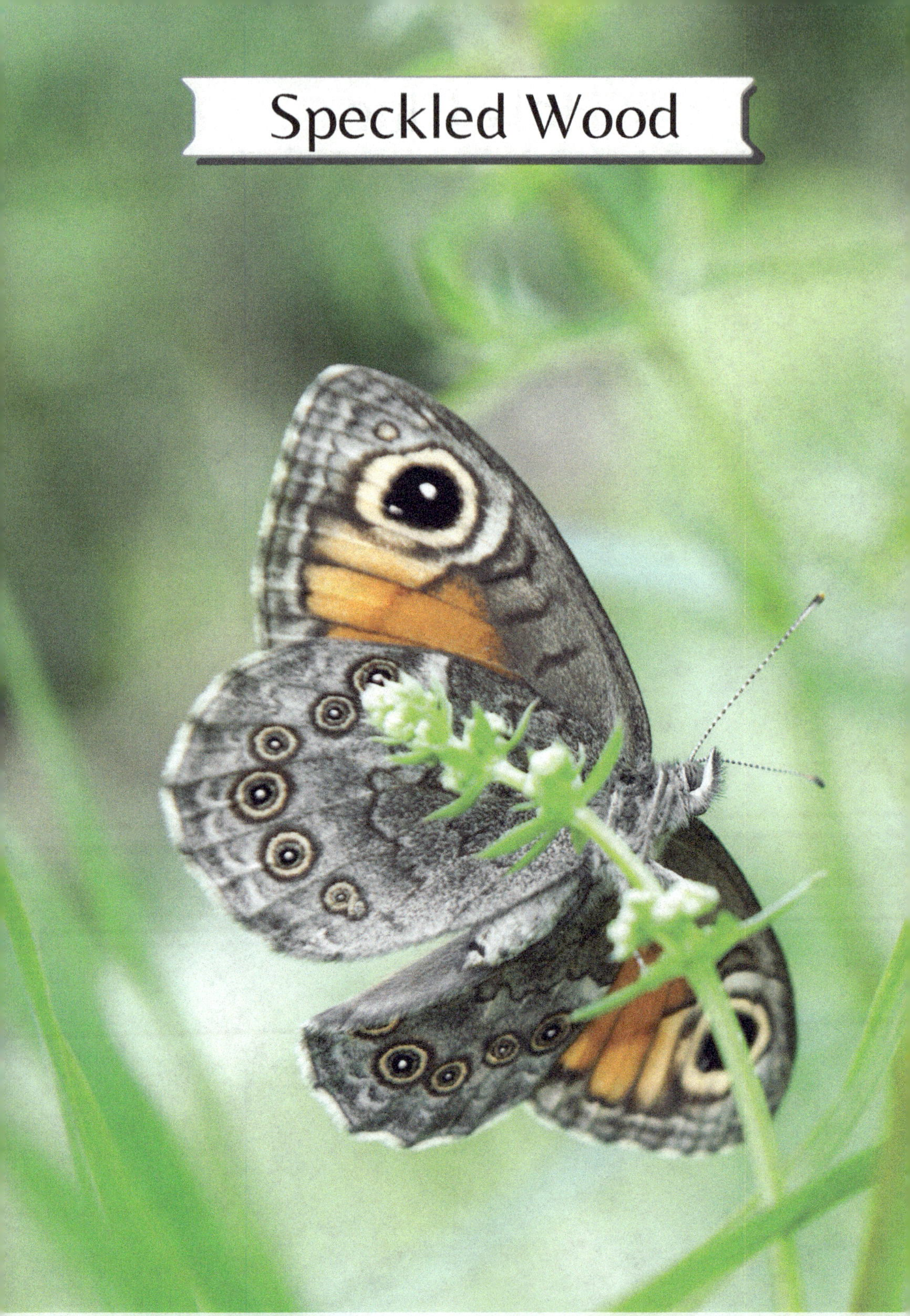

Like woodland light and often bask in sunbeams.

Meadow Brown

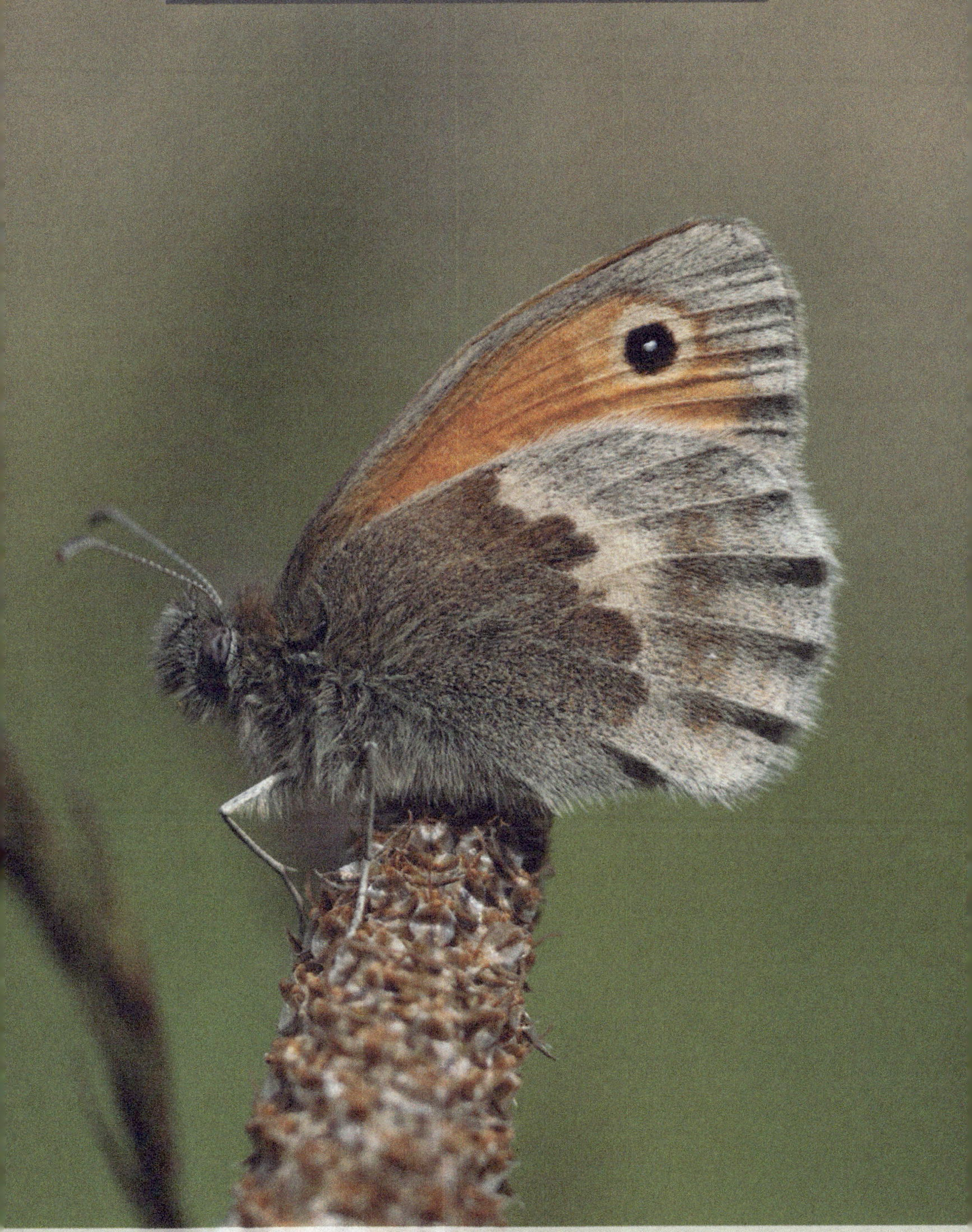

The most common butterfly in the UK.

Silver-Studded Blue

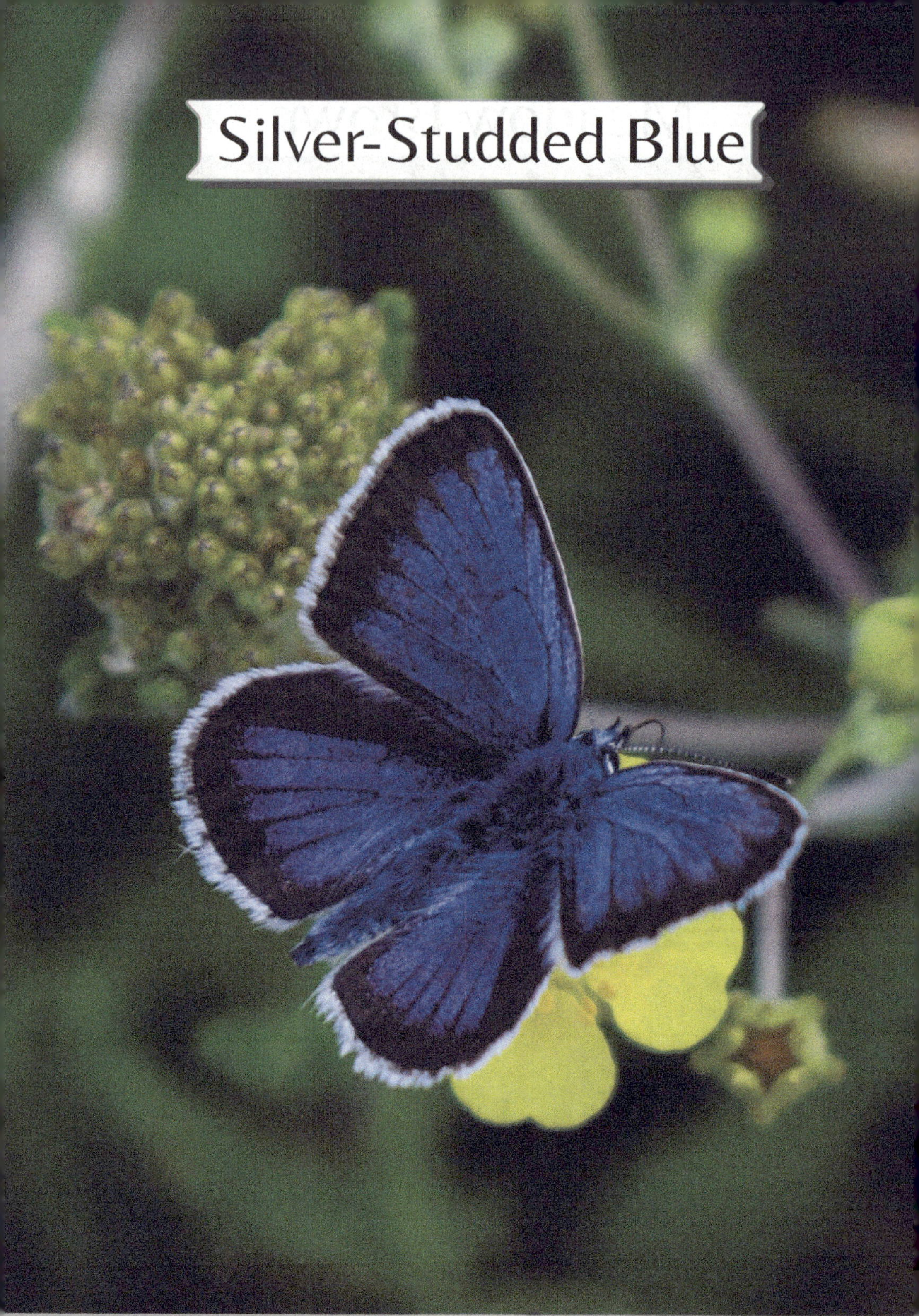

Fly in groups low over the heather.

Marsh Fritillary

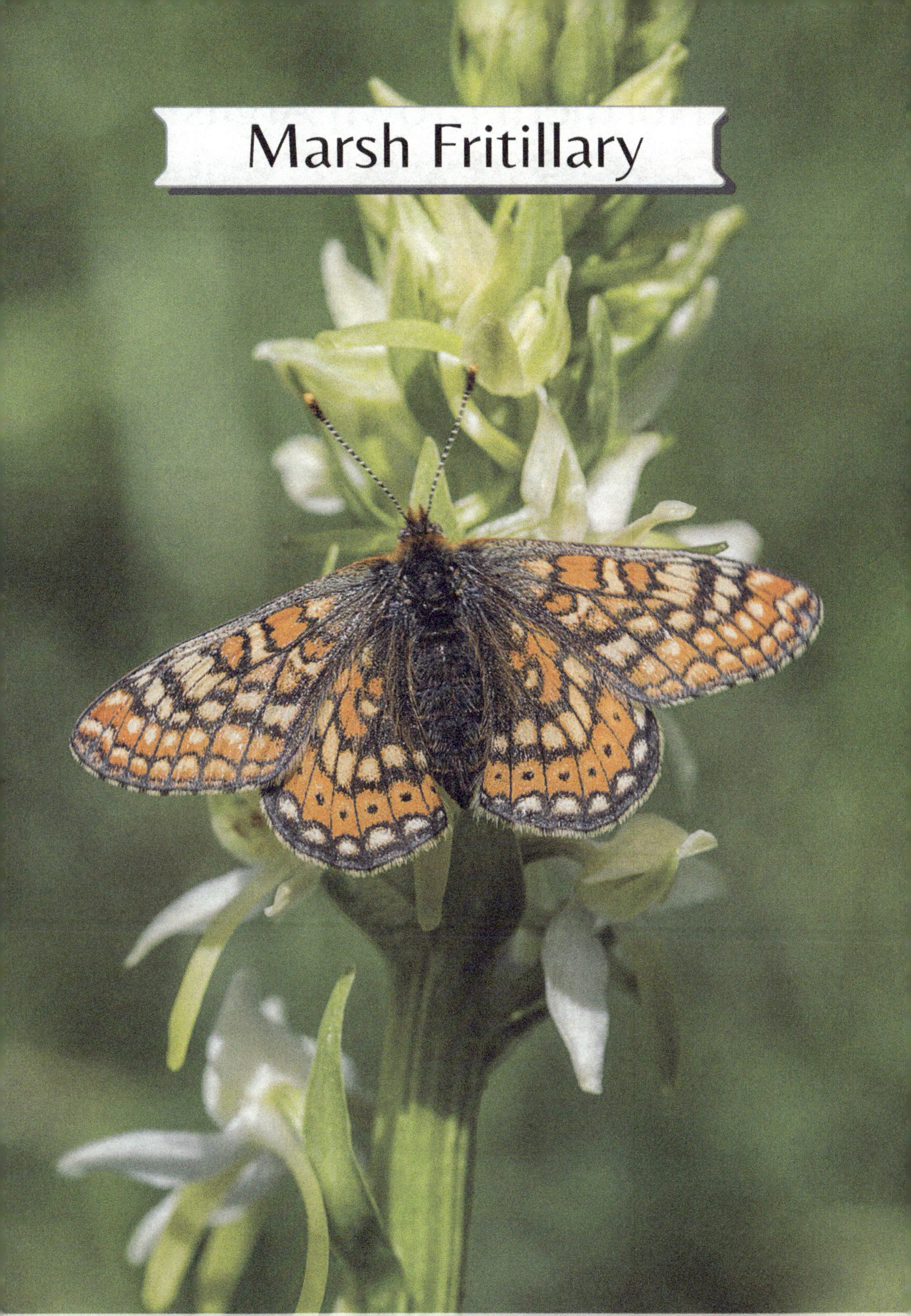

Found in damp grassland.

Northern Brown Argus

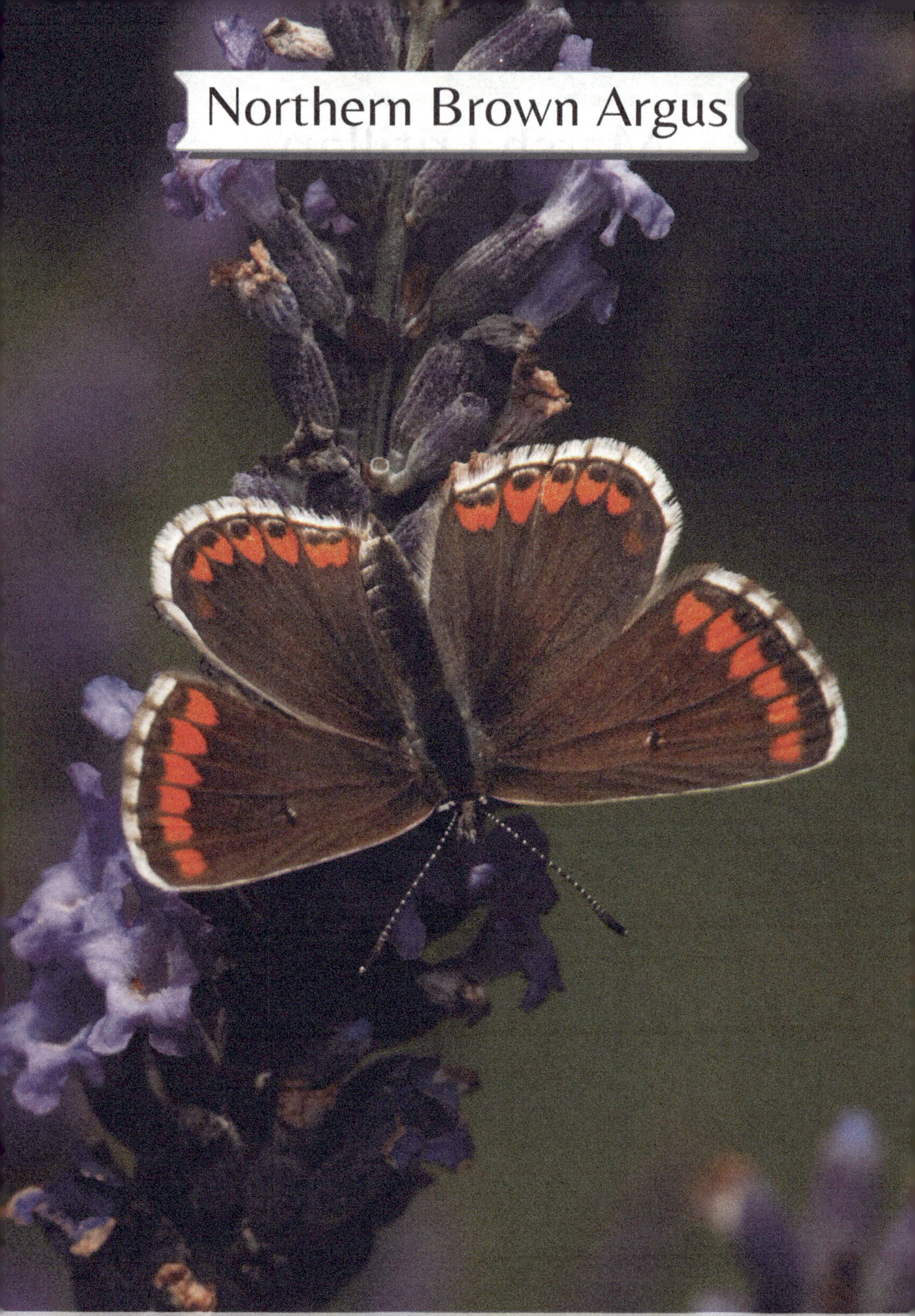

Mainly live in alpine and arctic places.

Painted Lady

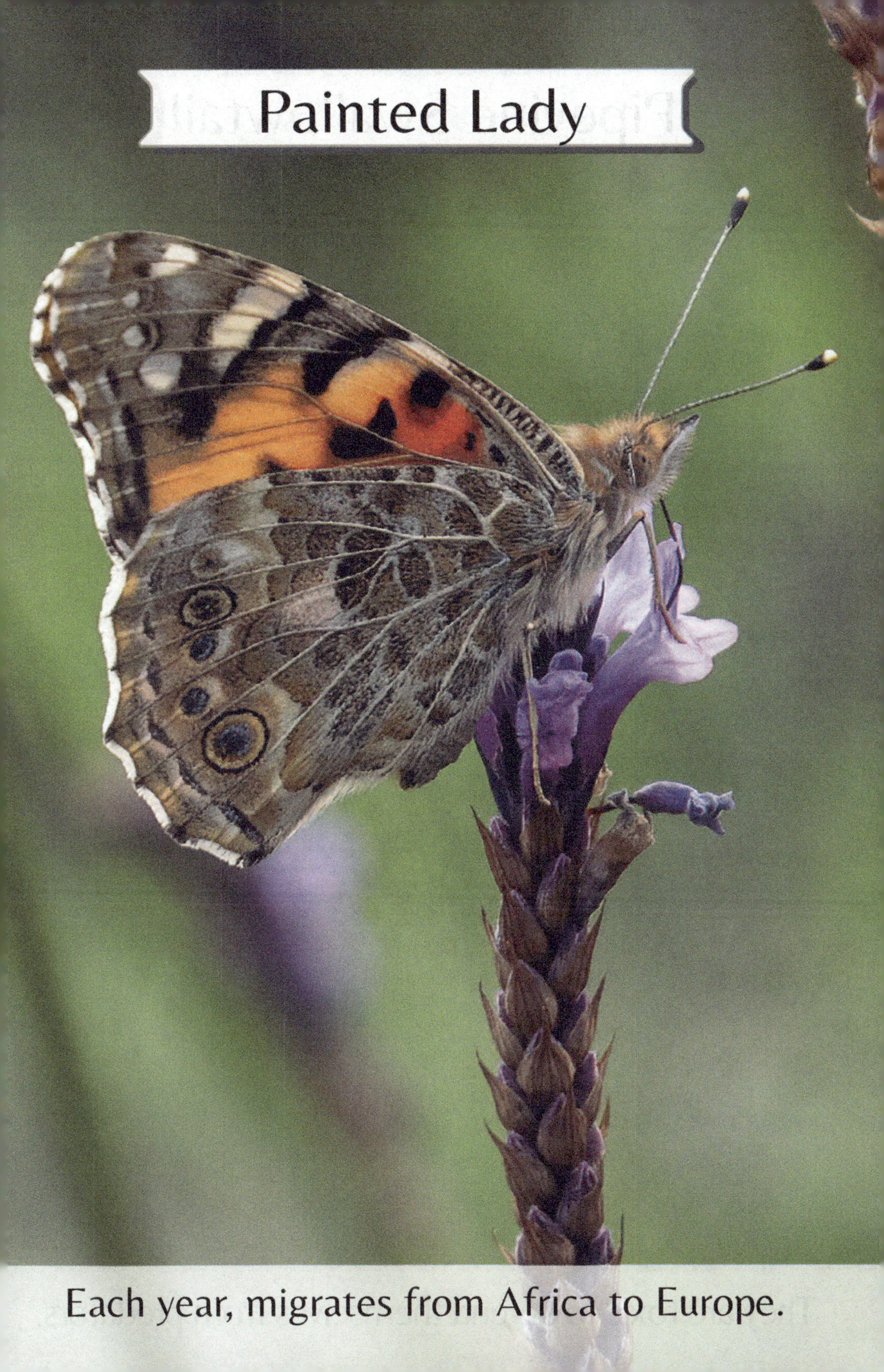

Each year, migrates from Africa to Europe.

Pipevine Swallowtail

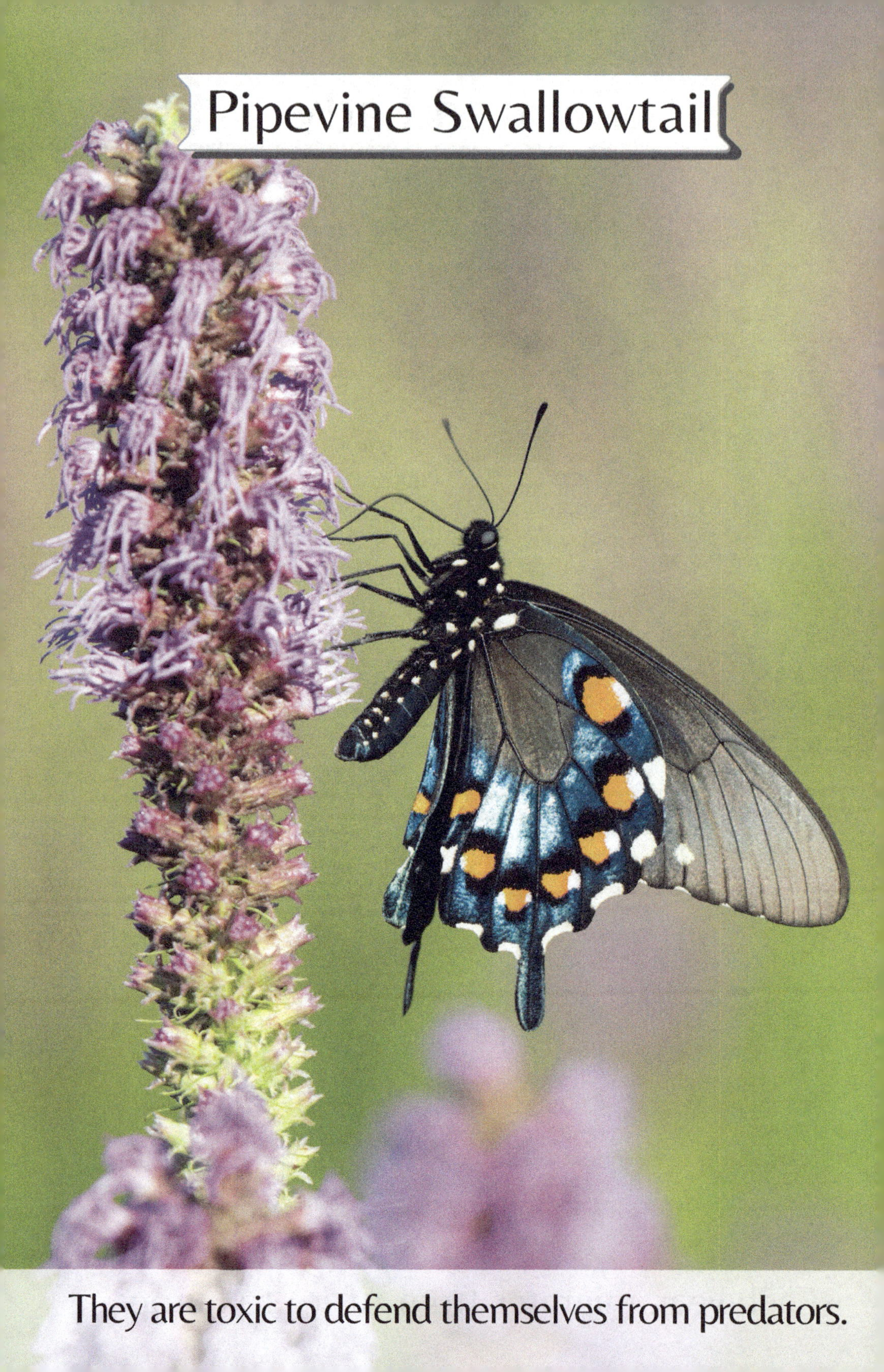

They are toxic to defend themselves from predators.

Peacock

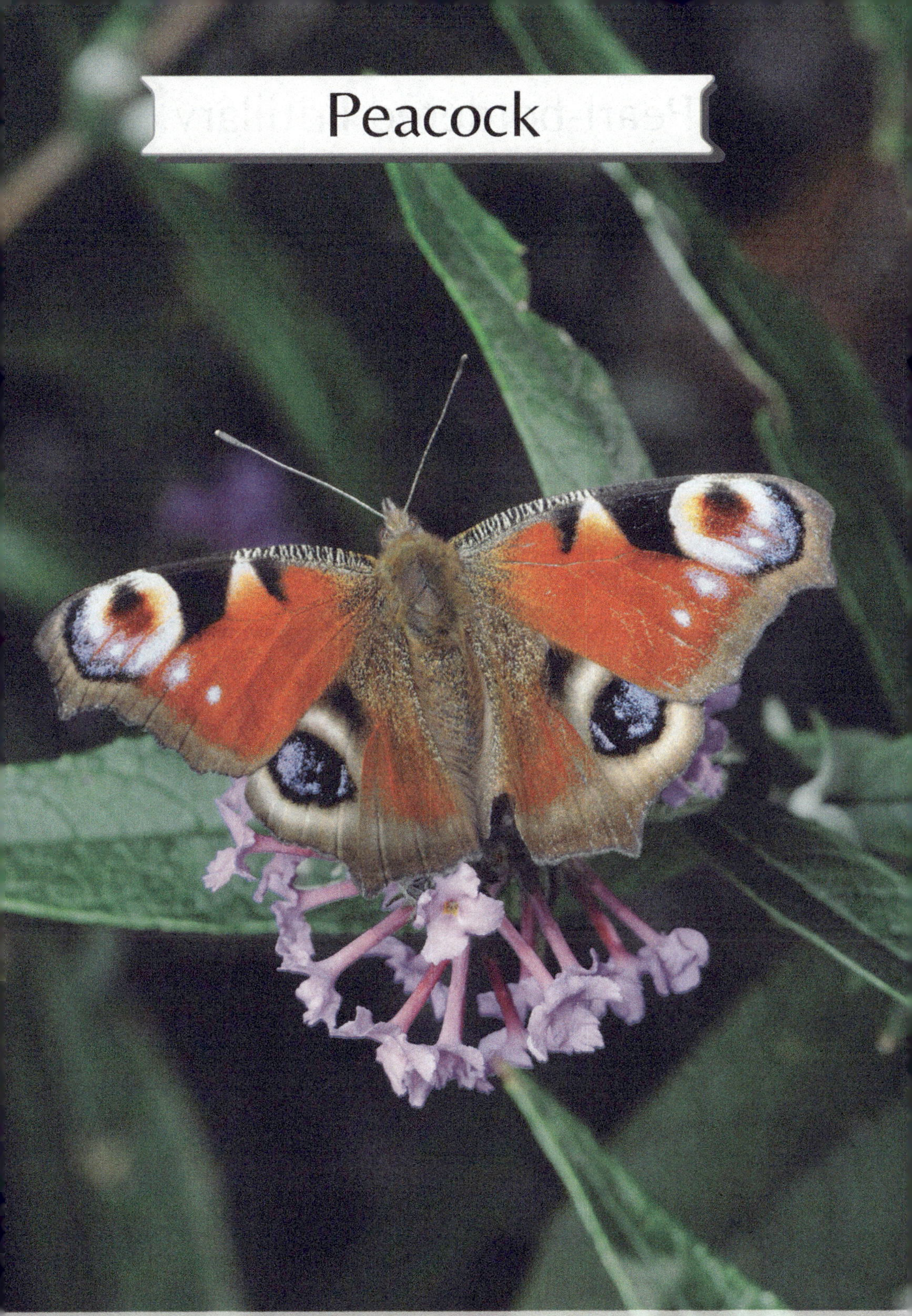

The eye-spots scare away birds and predators.

Pearl-bordered Fritillary

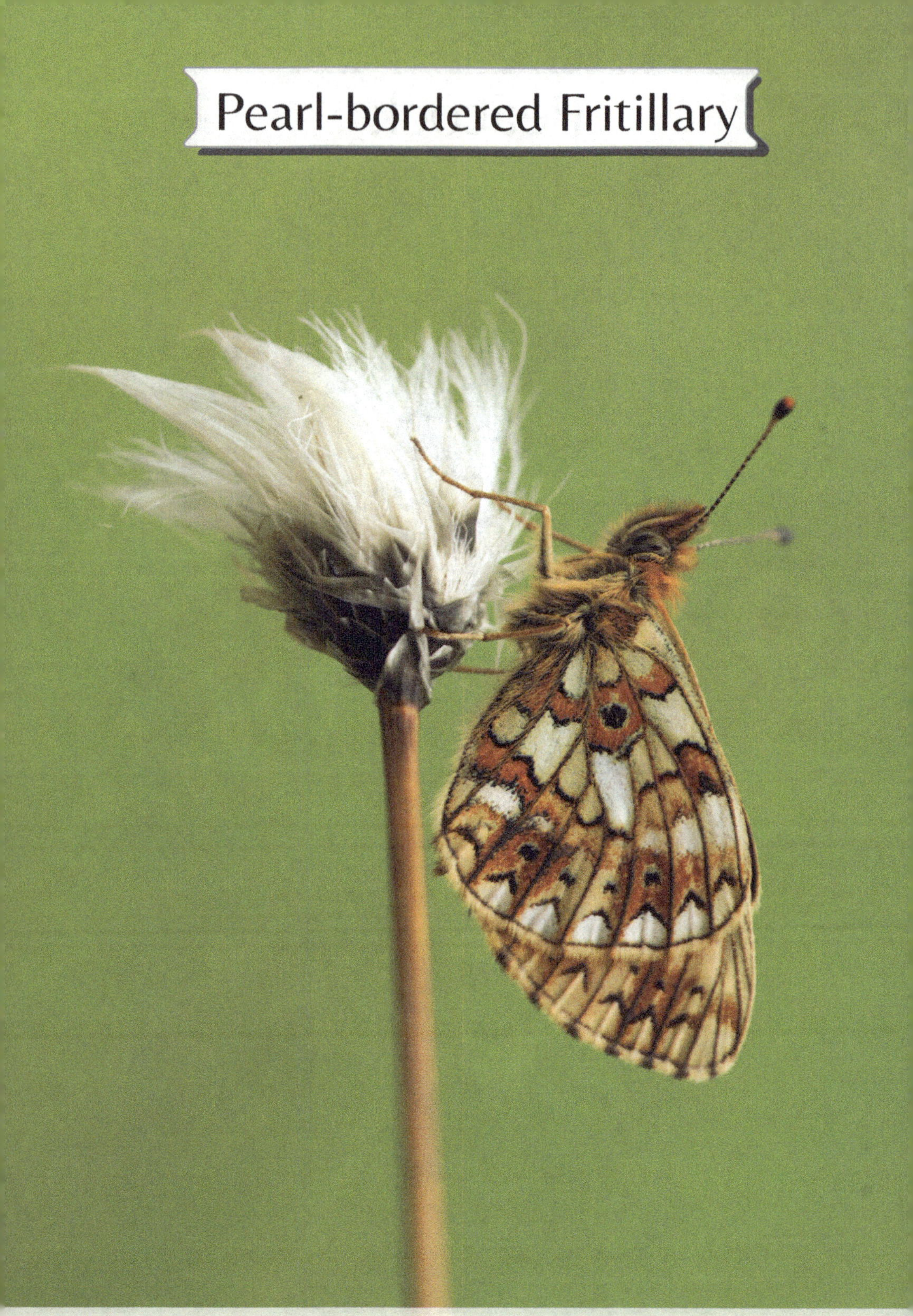

Named for its silvery 'pearl' spots.

Red Admiral

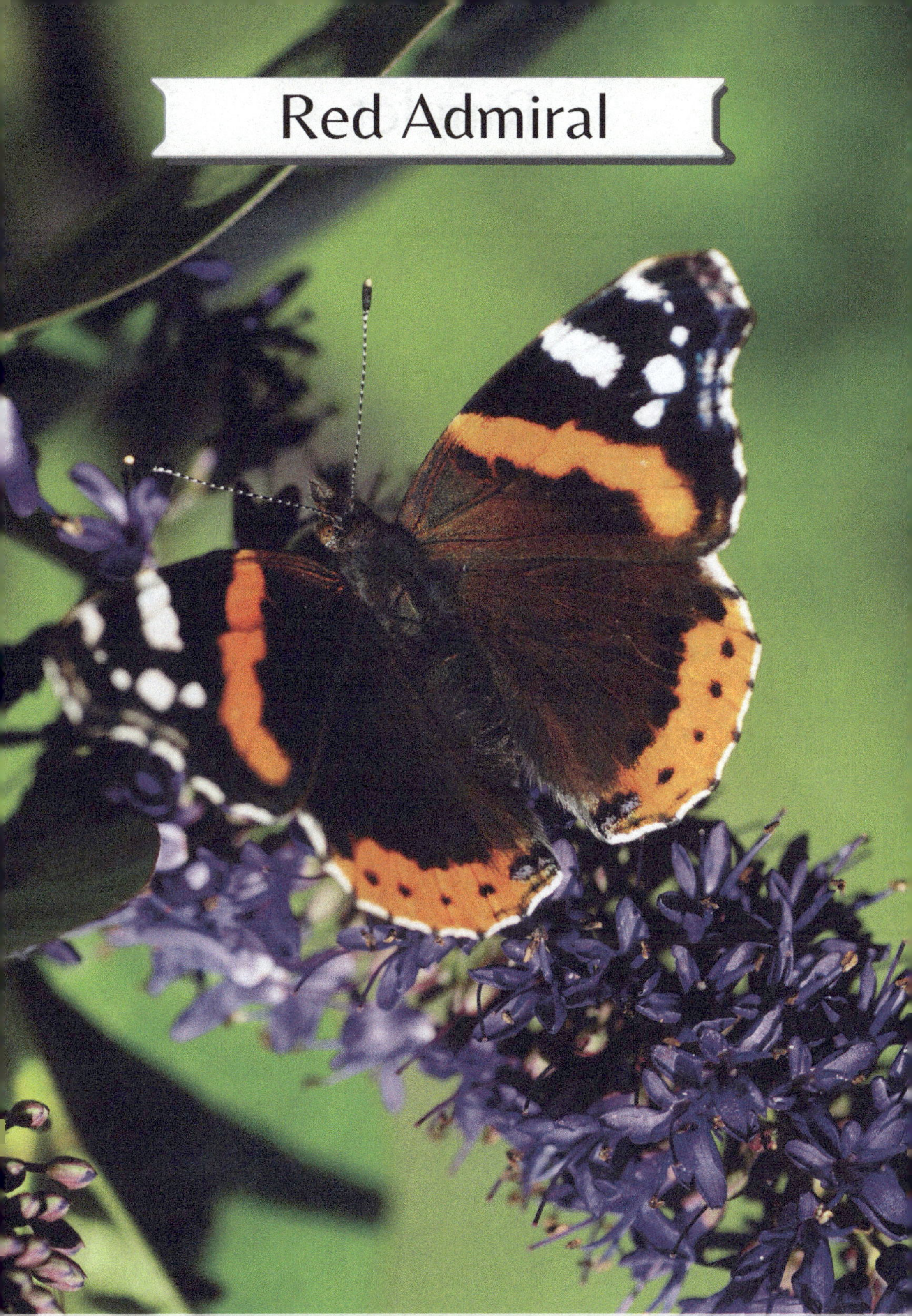

Known to love overripe fruit and nectar.

Ringlet

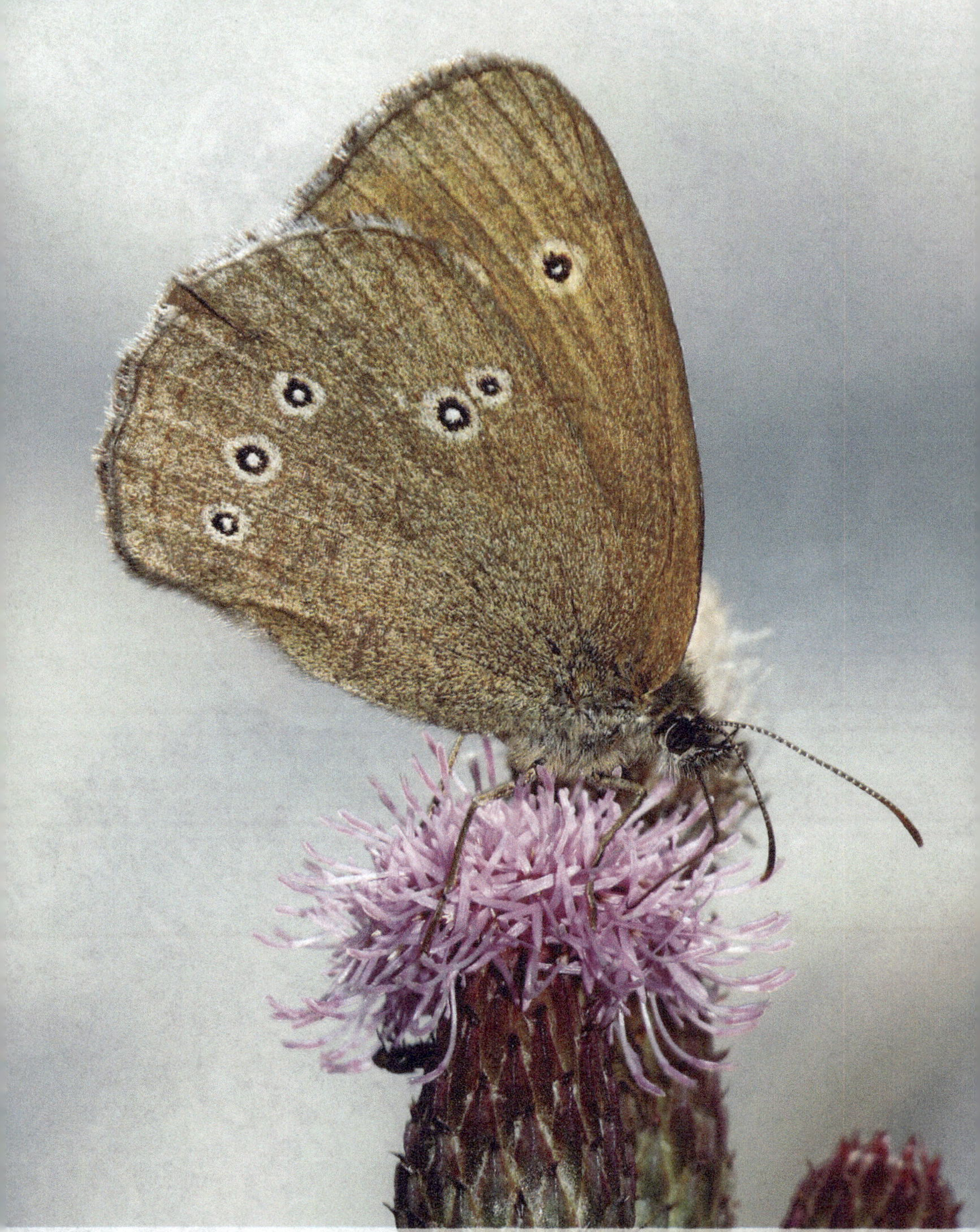

Named after the 'rings' on their wings.

Swallowtail

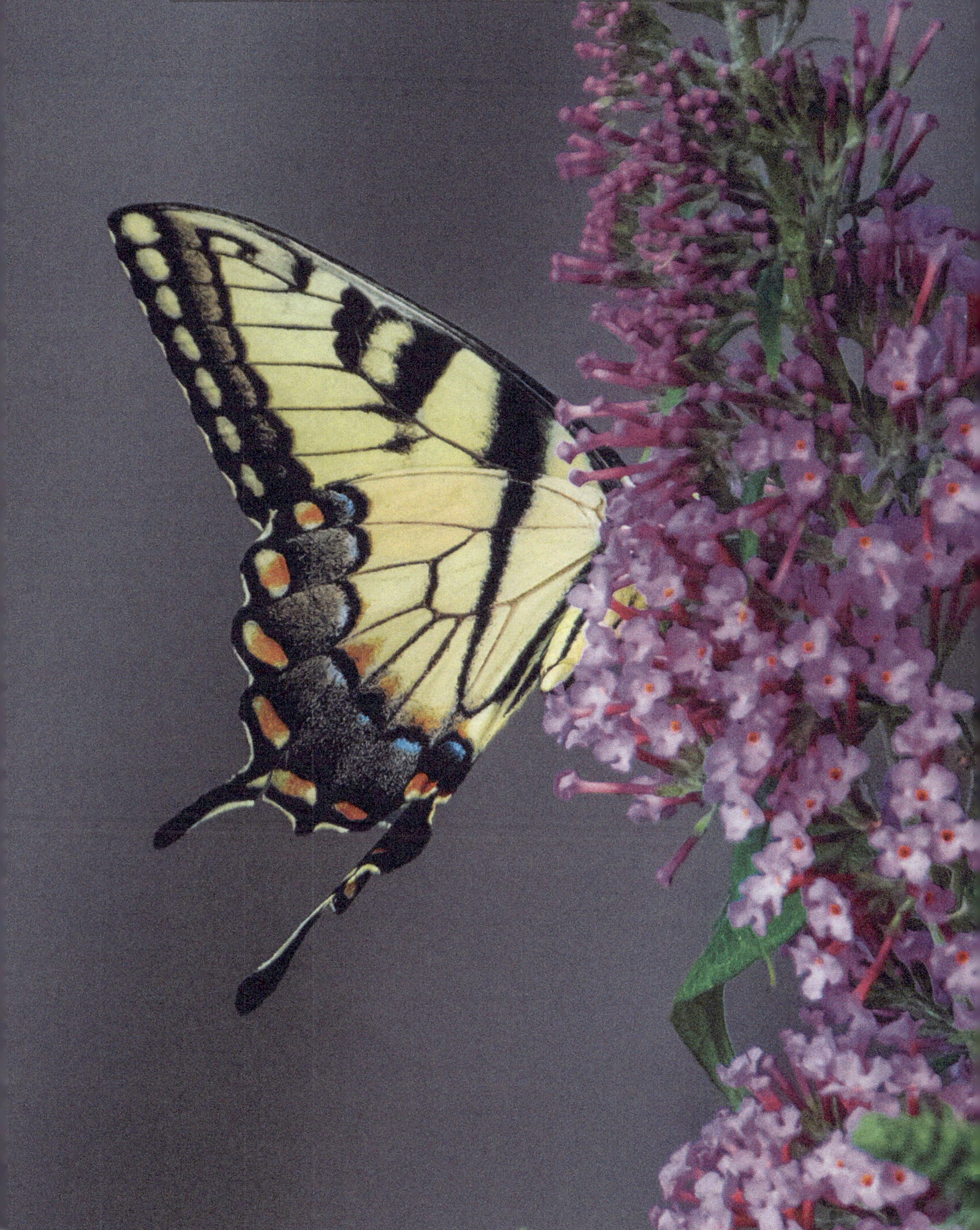

Their elegant tails resemble bird feathers.

Wood White

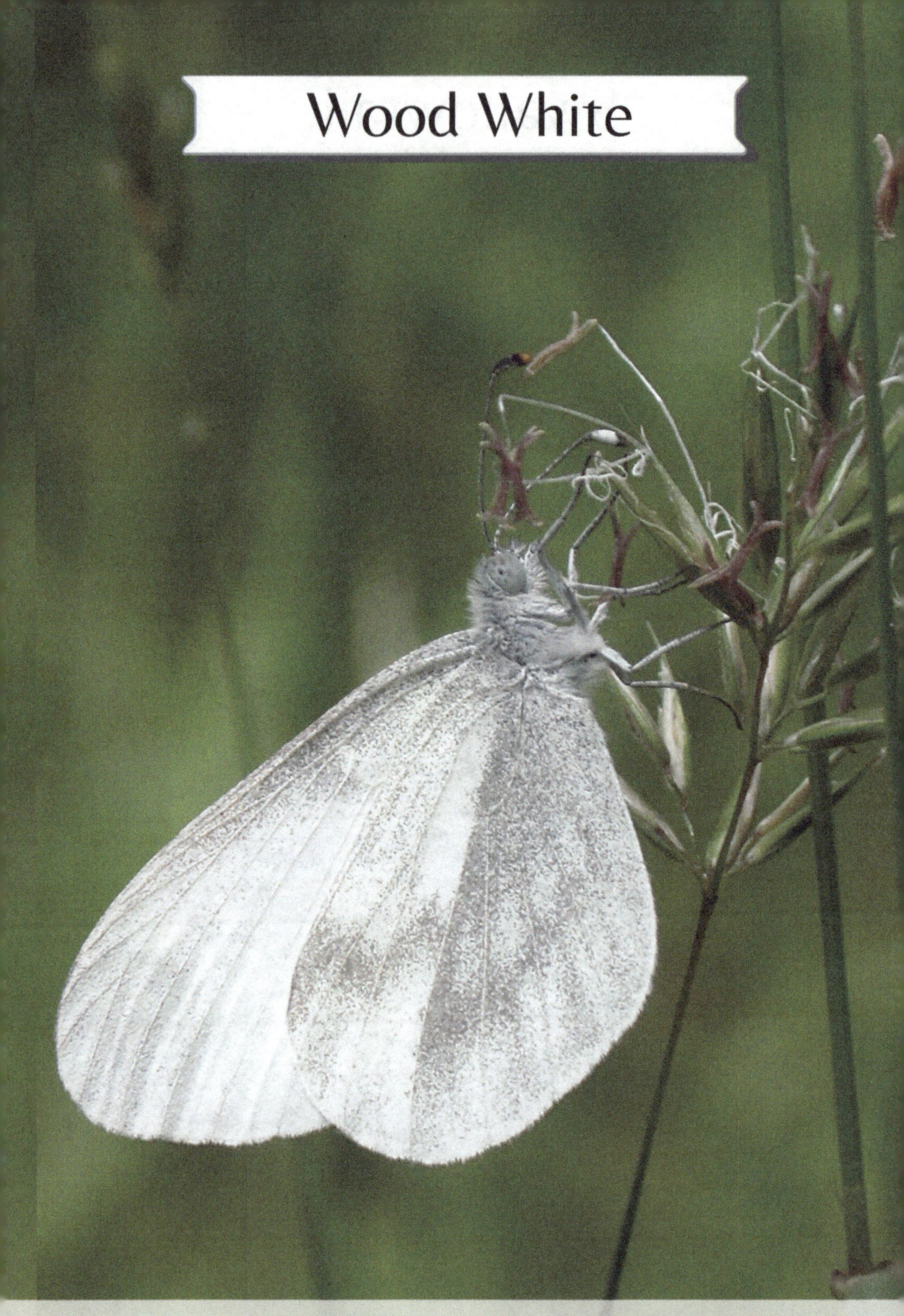

A weak flyer, that often flutters slowly.

White Admiral

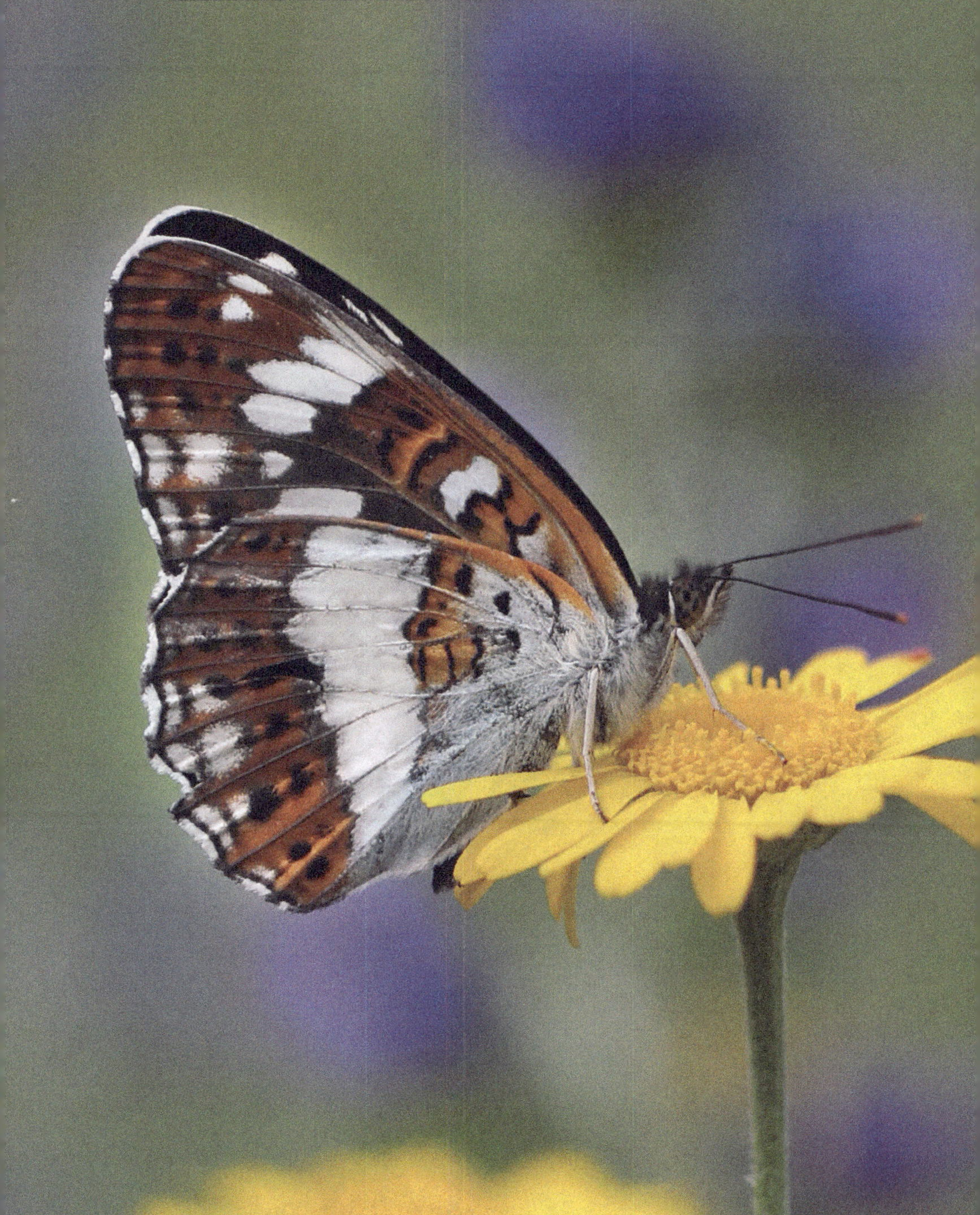

A graceful glider, found in woodlands.

Banded Orange

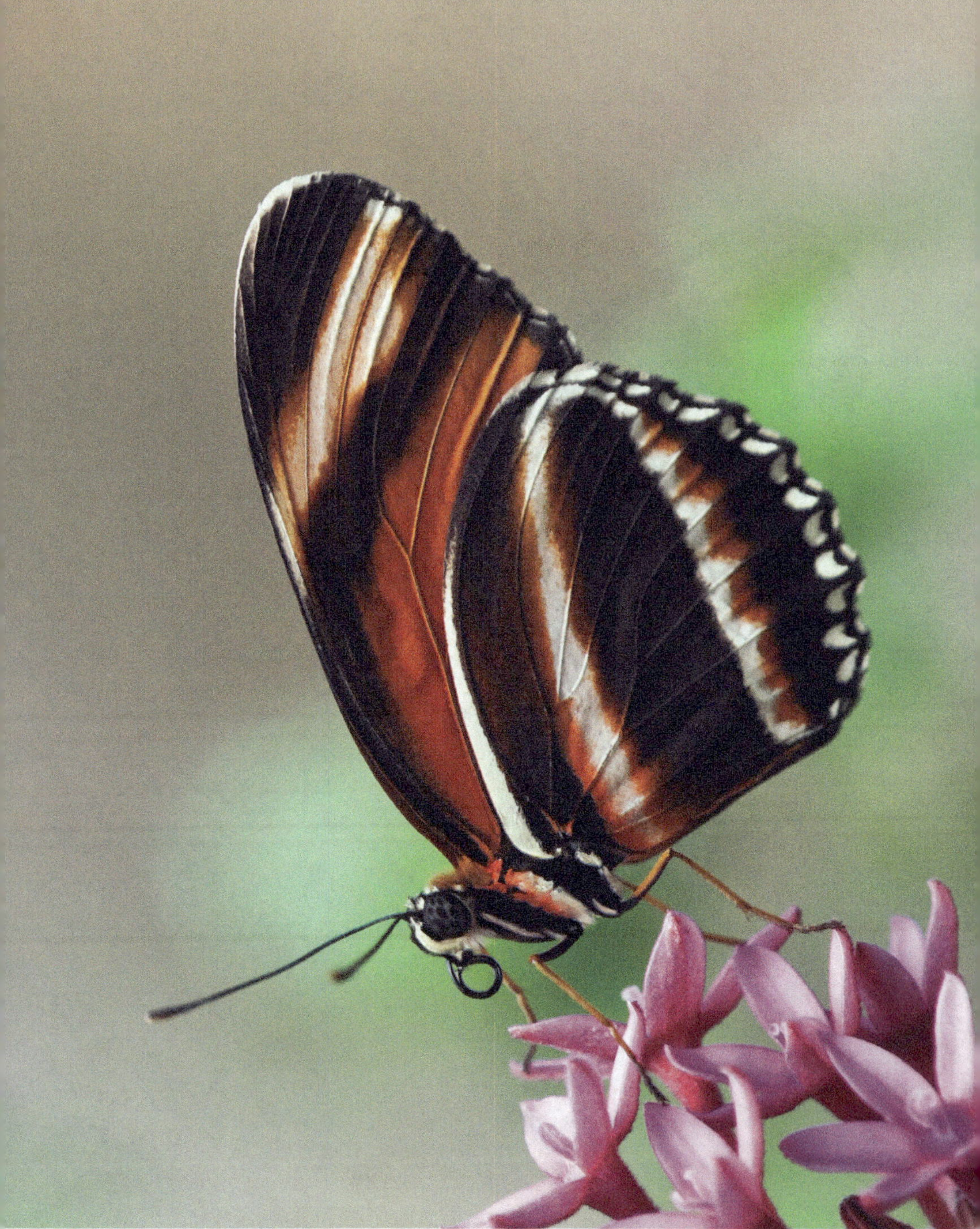

Also known as Orange Tiger.

Owl Butterfly

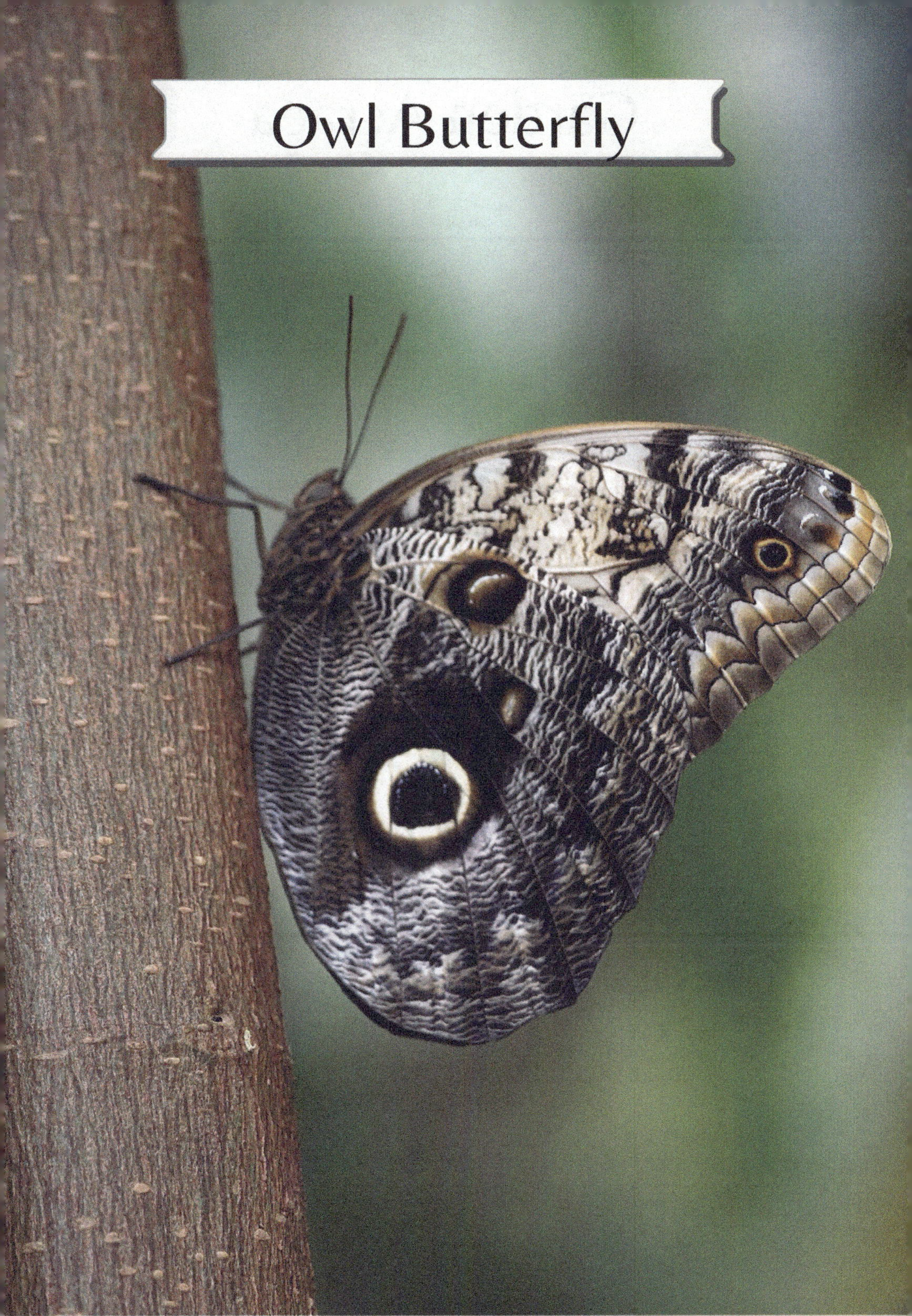

Its giant eye spots mimic owls to deter predators.

Garden Acraea

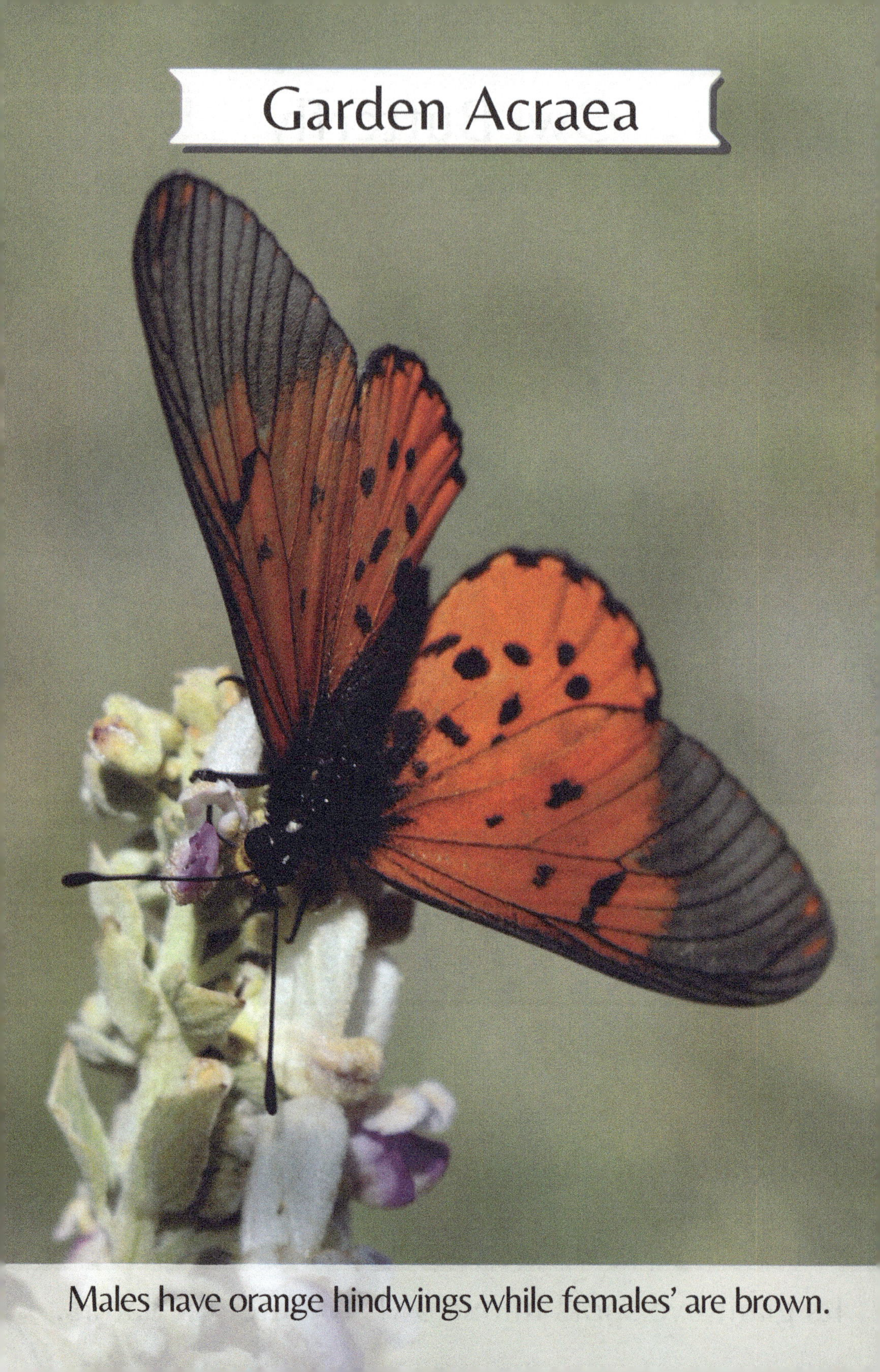

Males have orange hindwings while females' are brown.

Glasswing

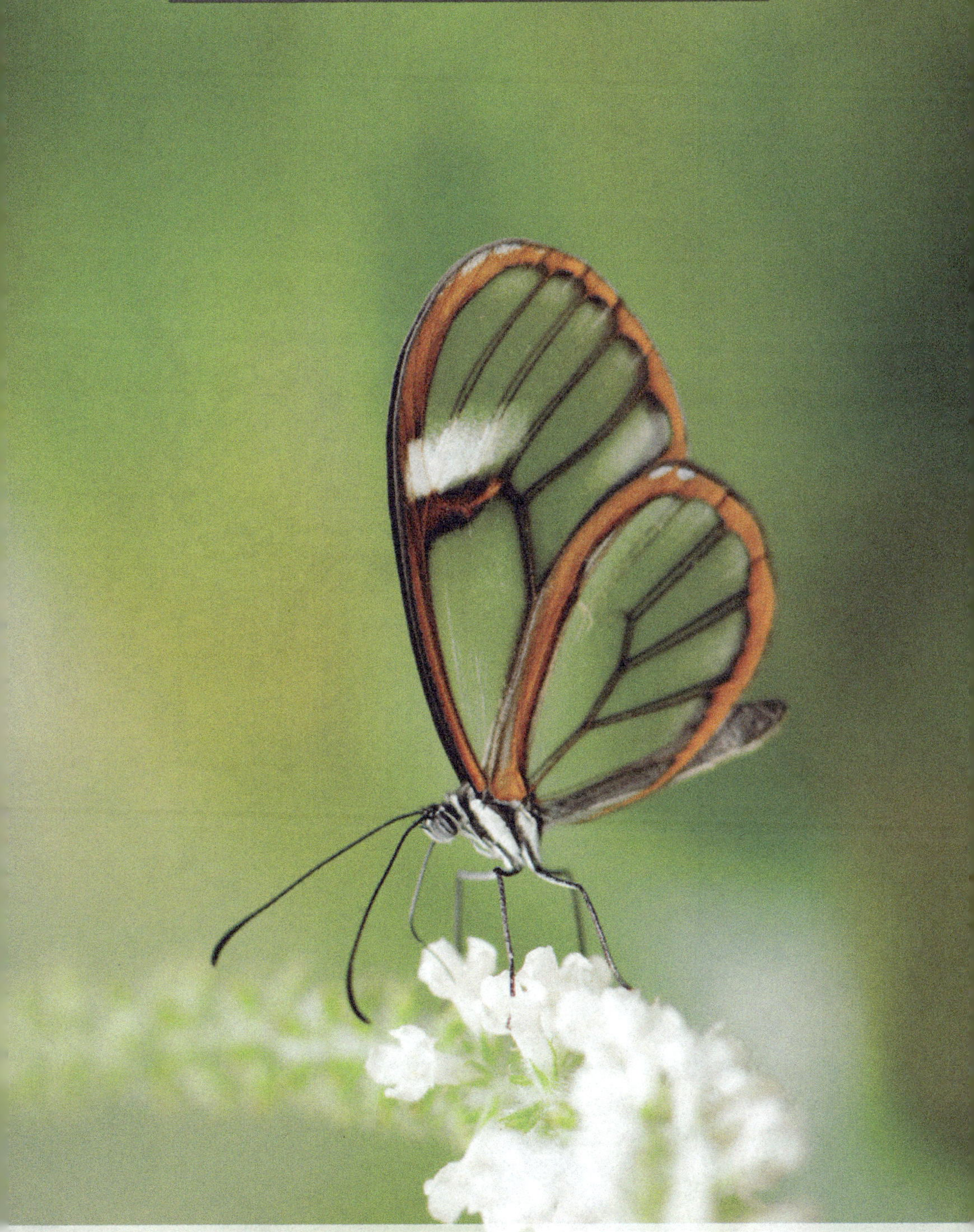

The wings look like clear glass!

Spicebush Swallowtail

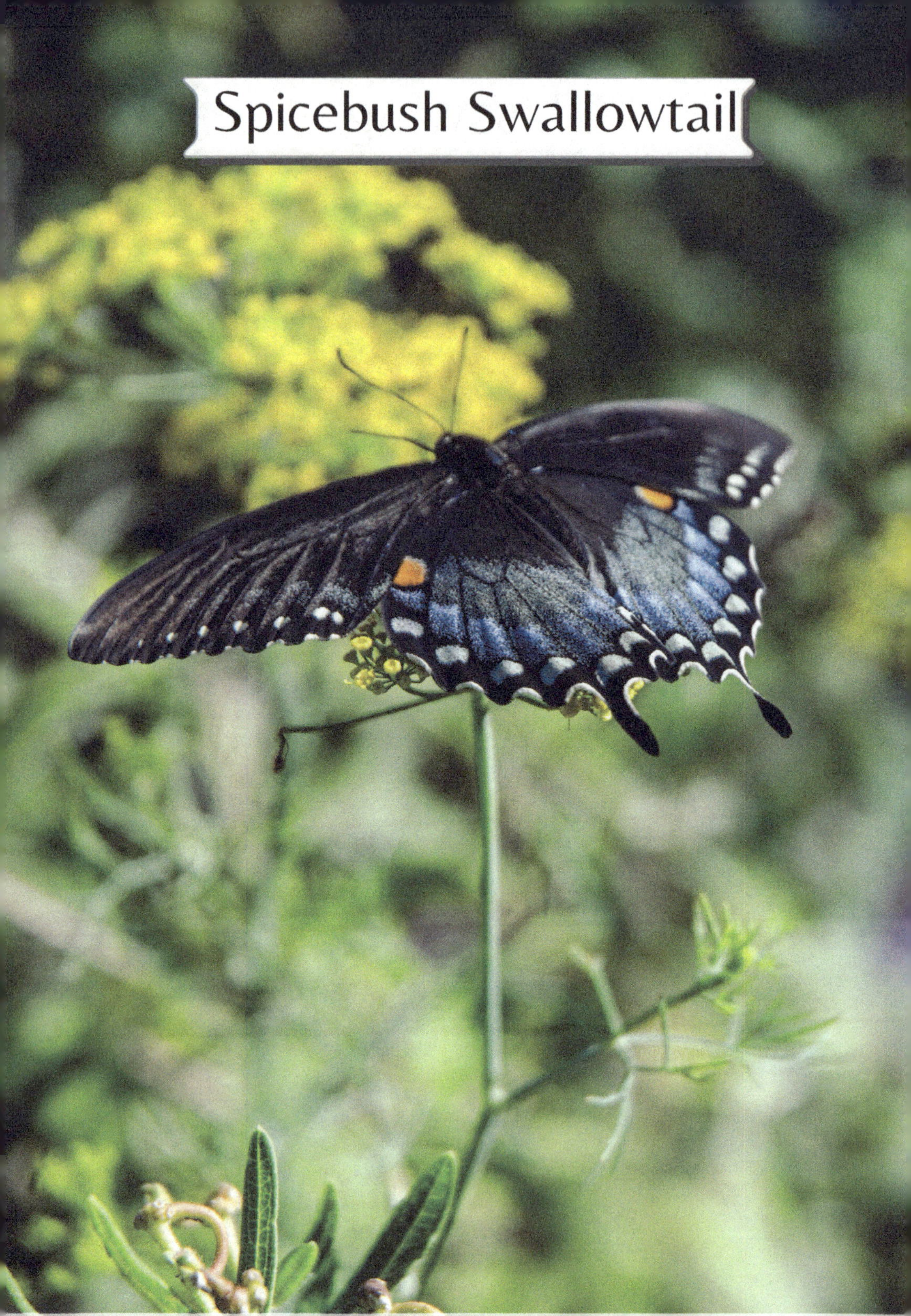

Looks like toxic butterflies for protection.

Leafwing

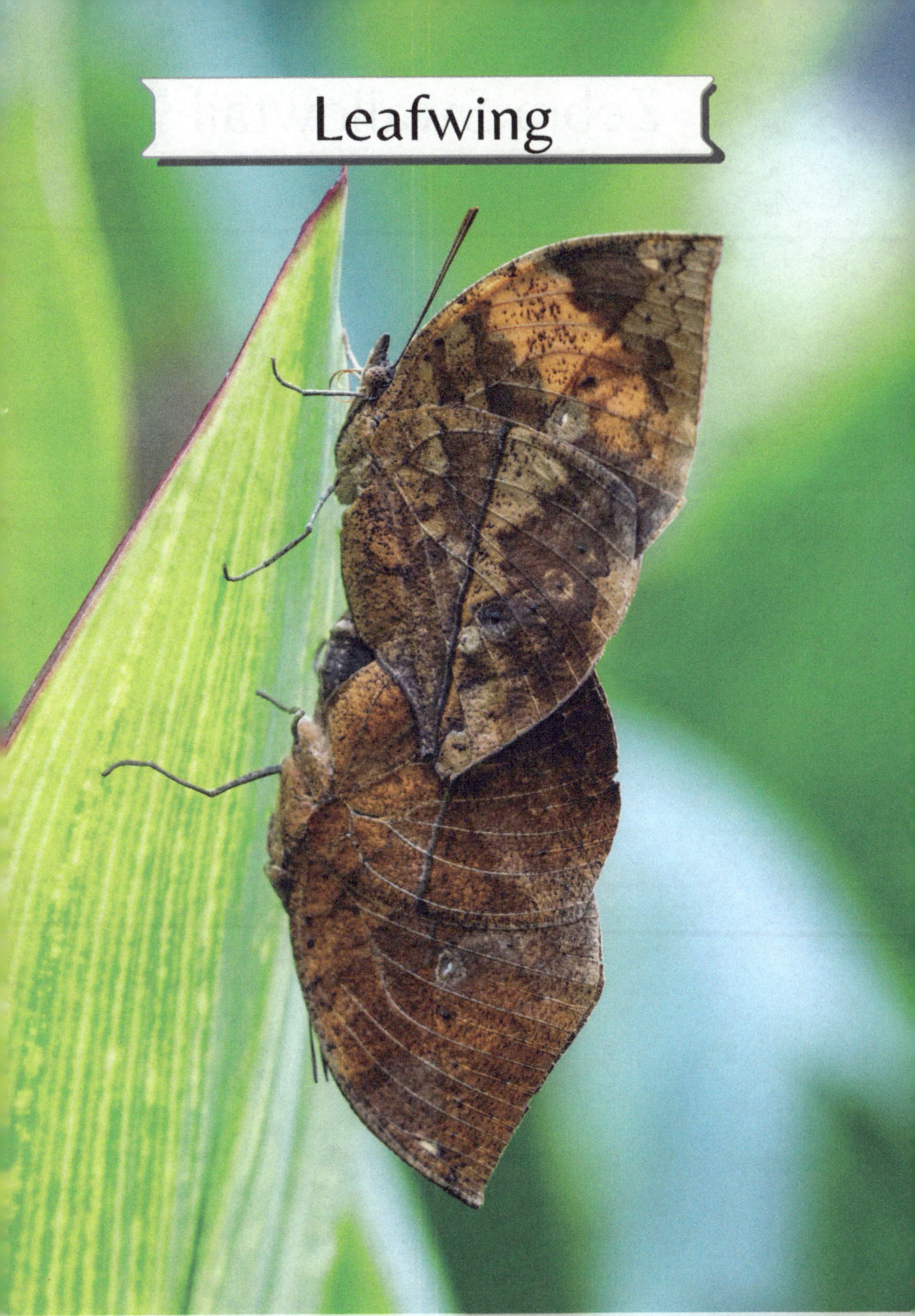

Leafwings can camouflage perfectly as leaves!

Zebra Swallowtail

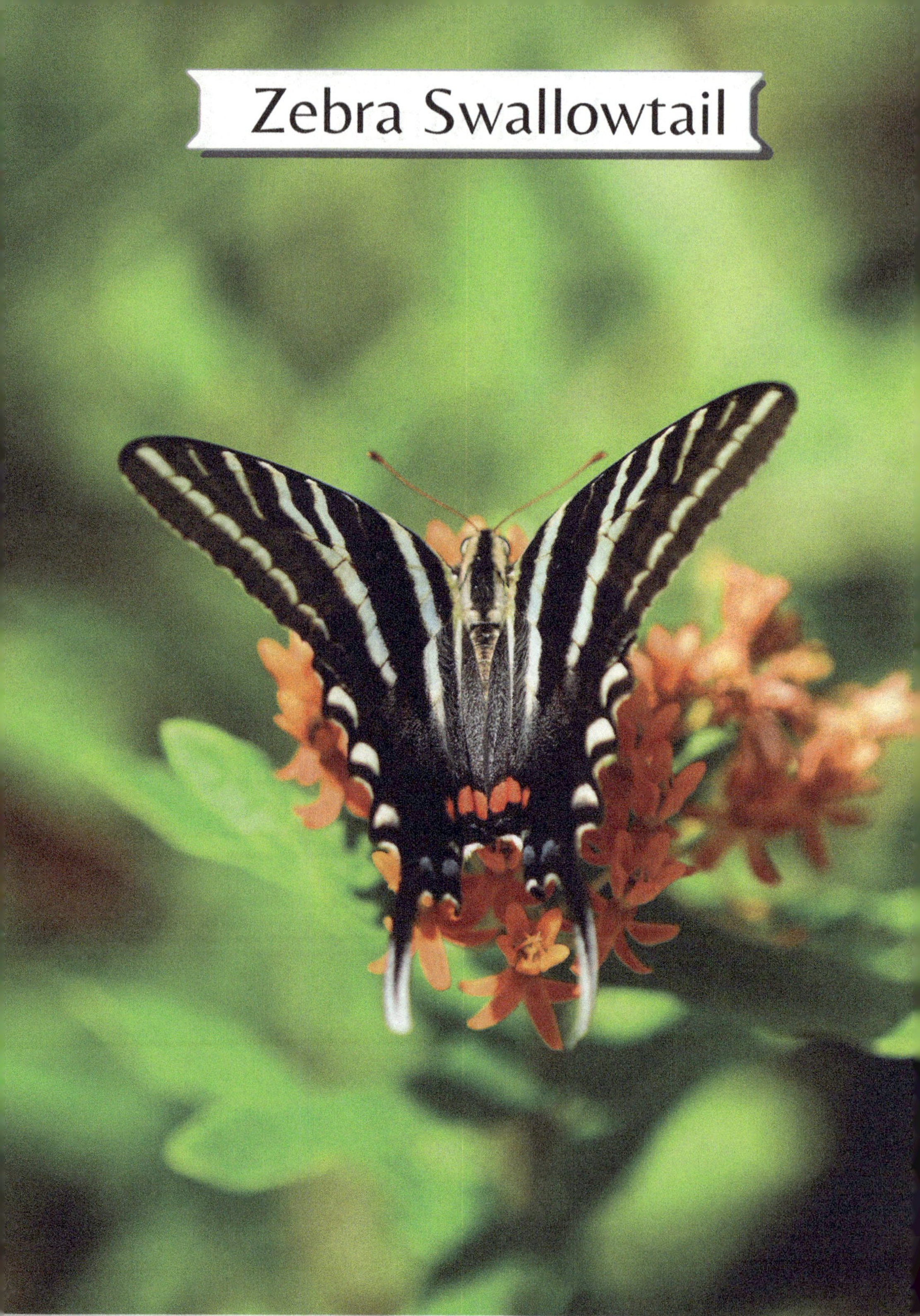

Known to have the longest tail of any butterfly!

Great Spangled Fritillary

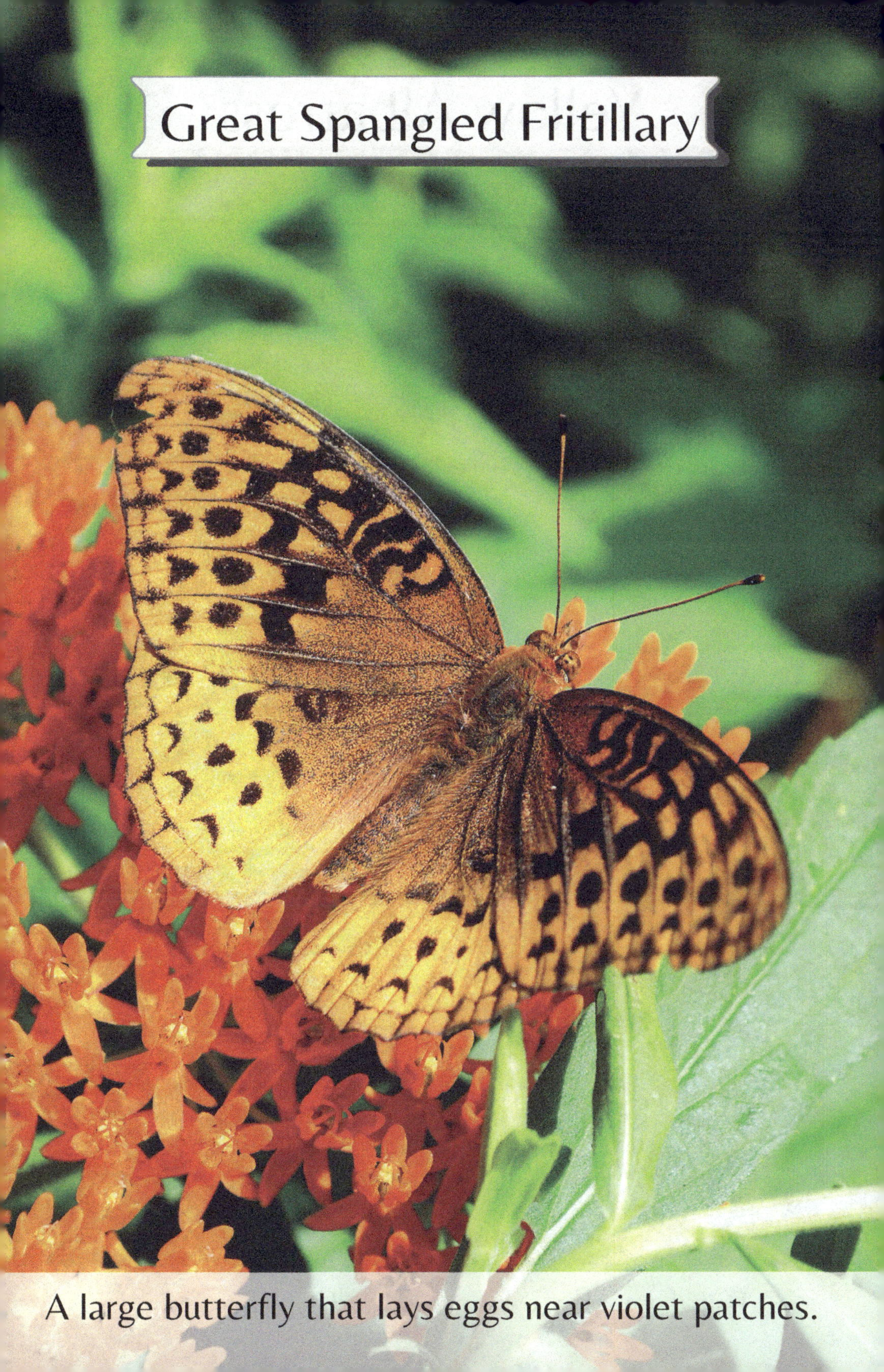

A large butterfly that lays eggs near violet patches.

Yellow Albatross

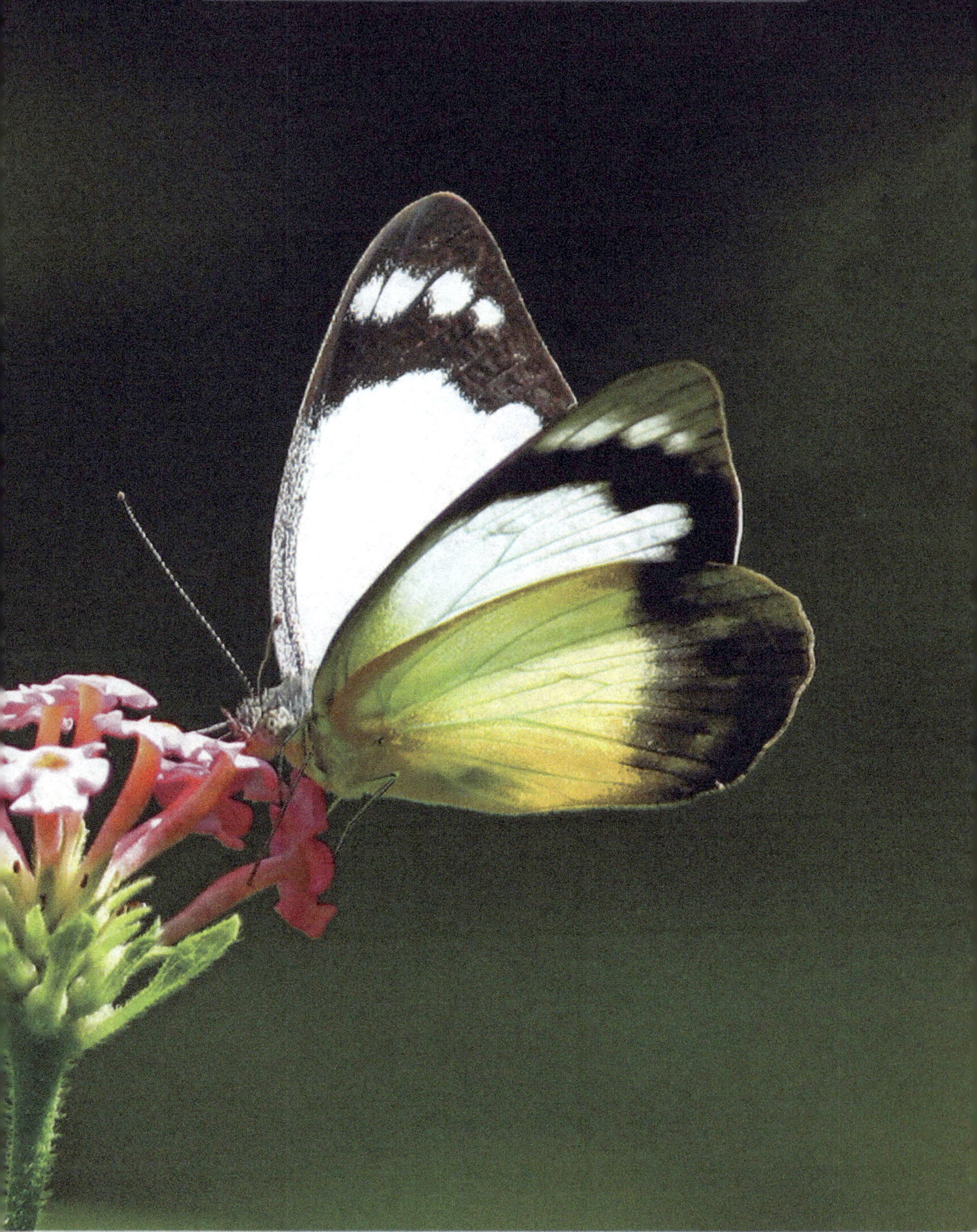

Bright yellow butterfly that flies fast!

Striped Albatross

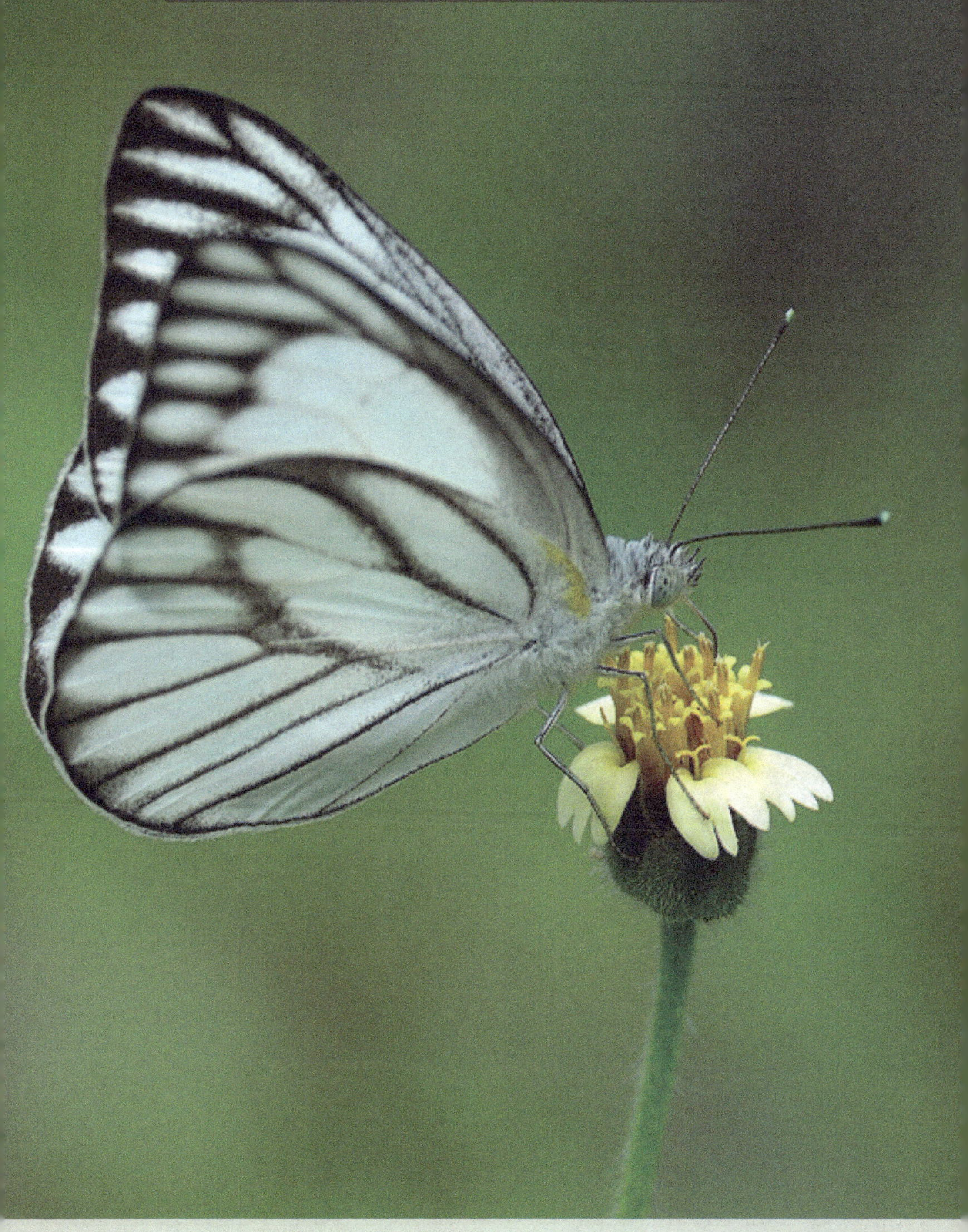

A rare species originating from India and Sri Lanka.

Pea Blue

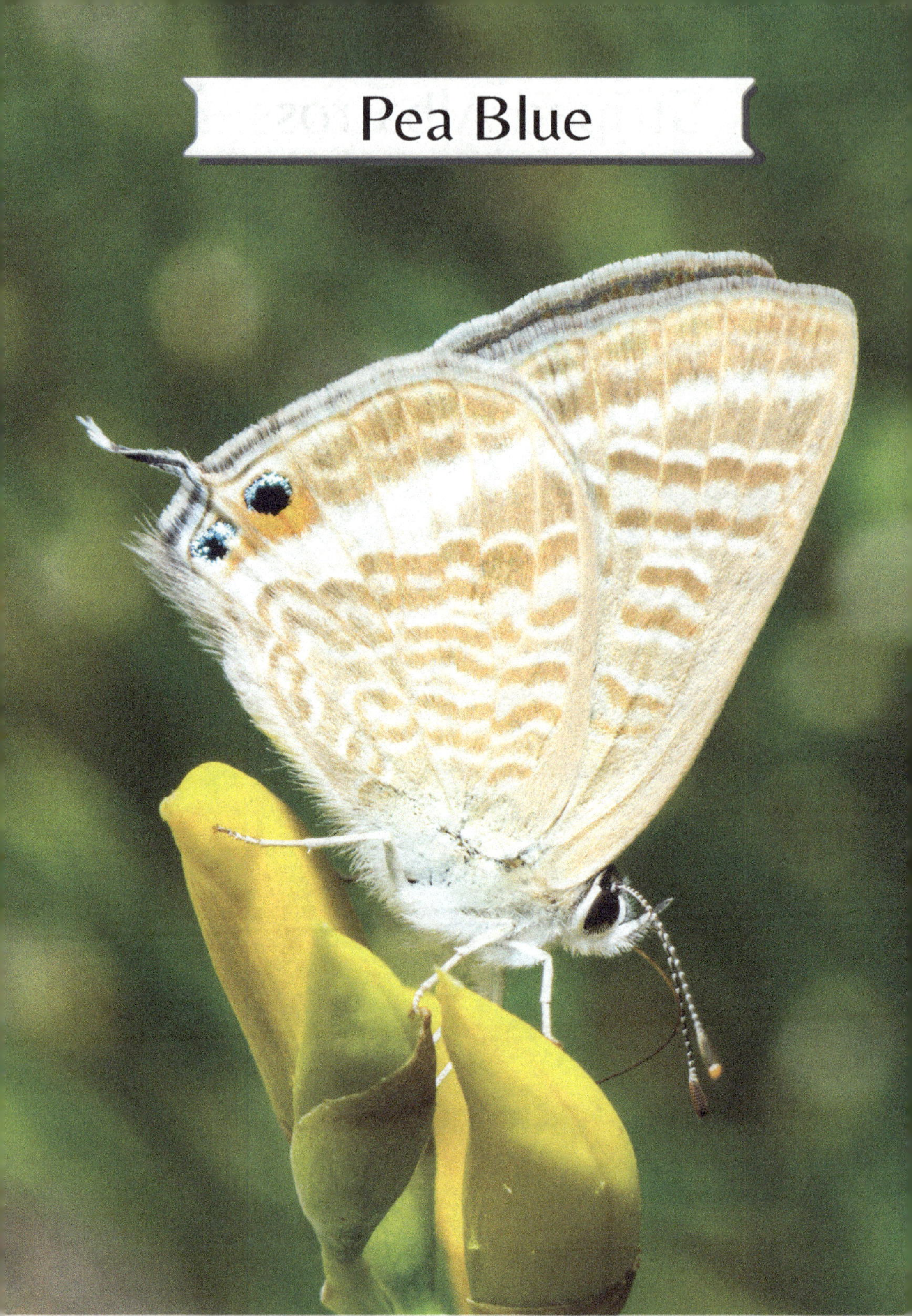

A tiny butterfly with tail streamers.

Eastern Bath White

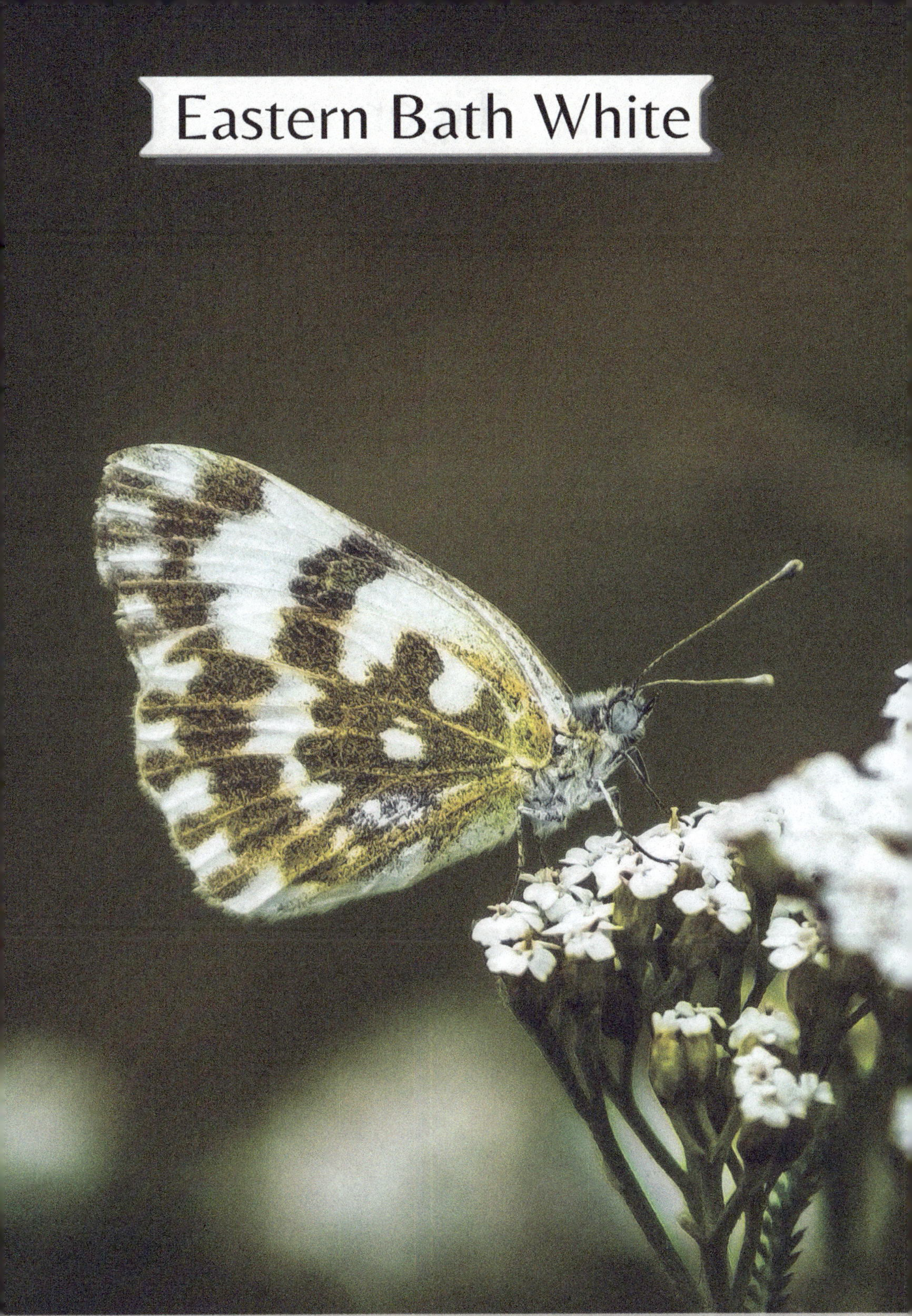

Their underwings have green marbled patterns.

Tiger

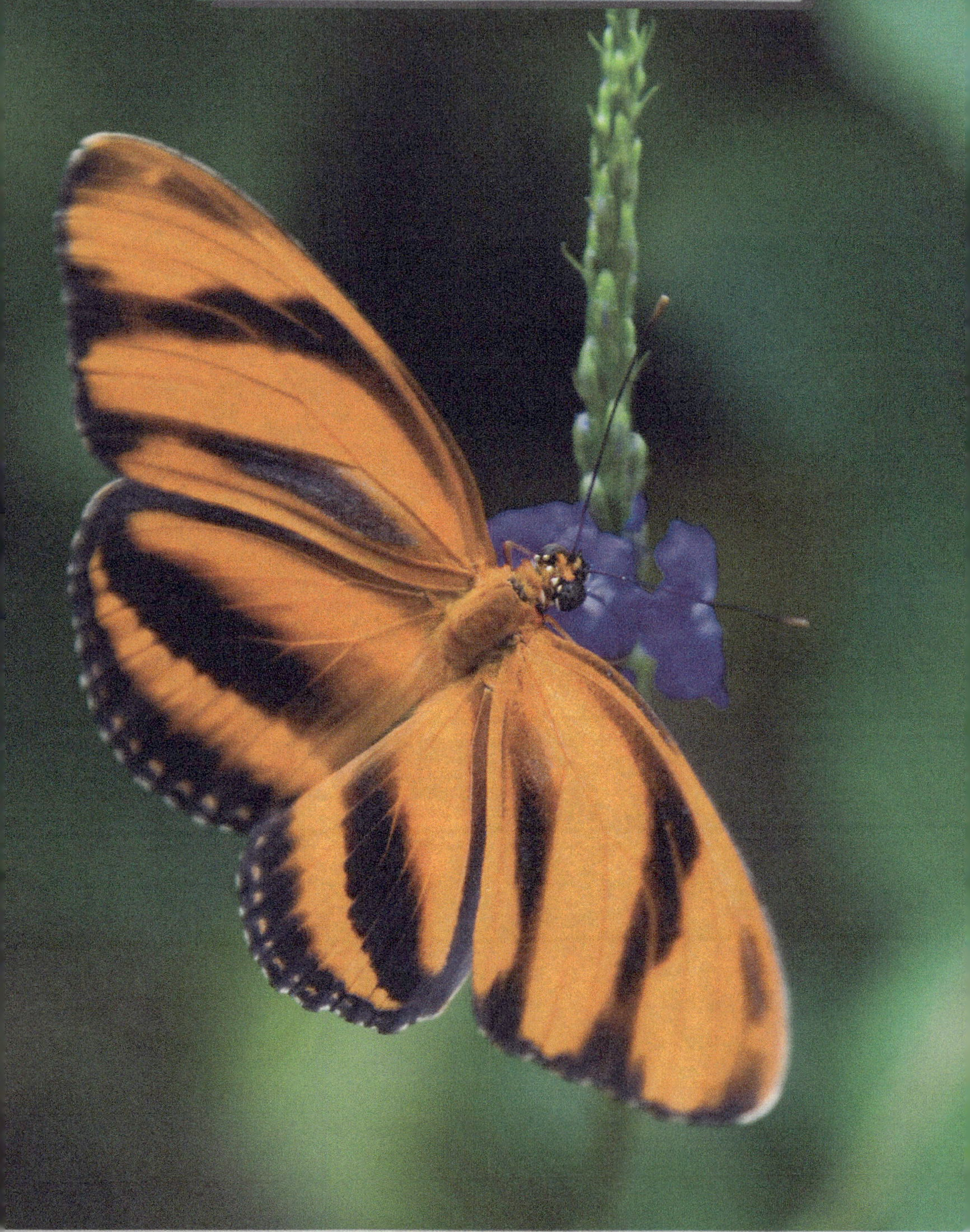

The tiger stripes actually scare away predators.

Mourning Cloak

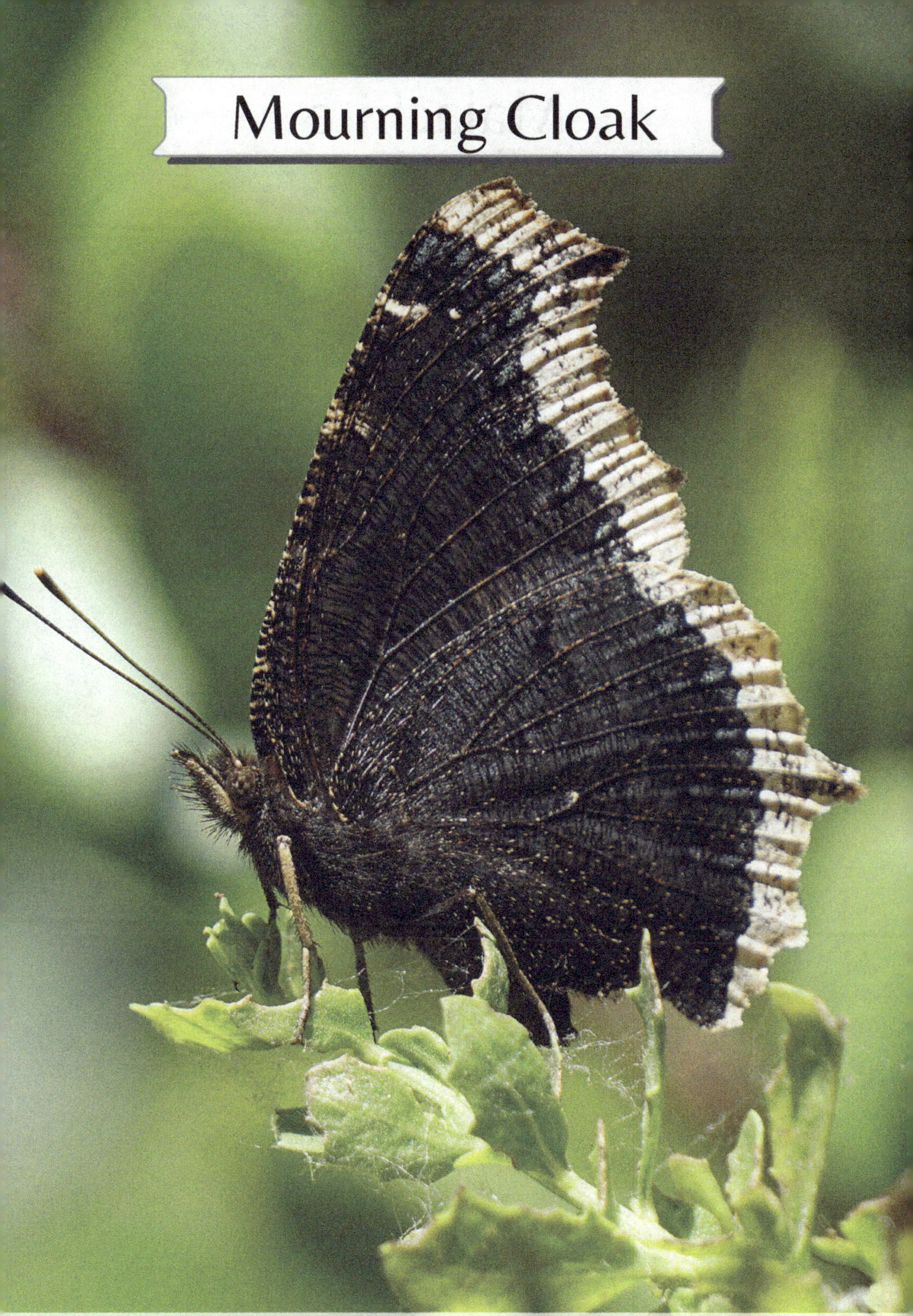

Can live for nearly a year (a long butterfly lifespan)!

Malachite

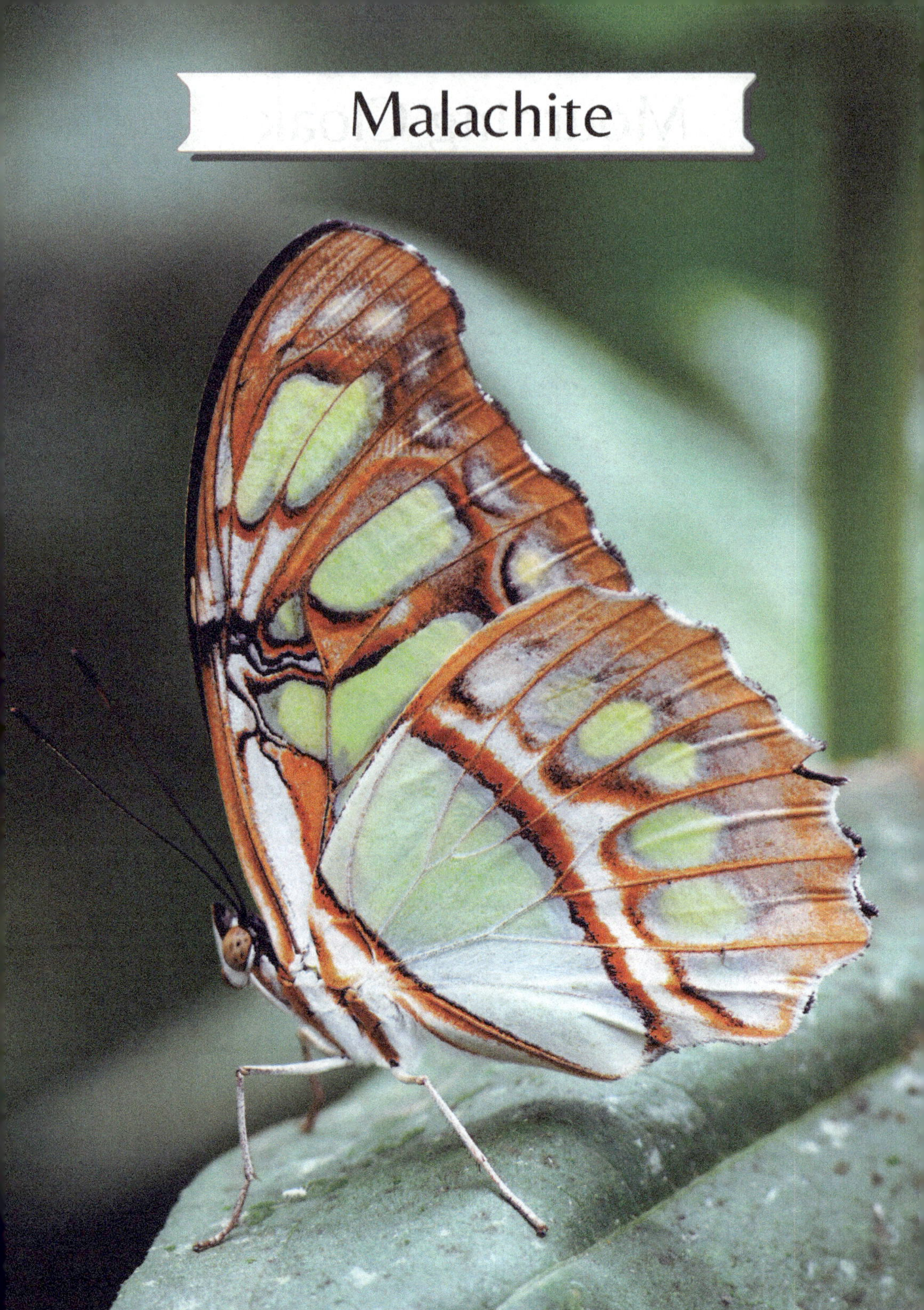

Named after the green gemstone malachite.

Blue Pansy

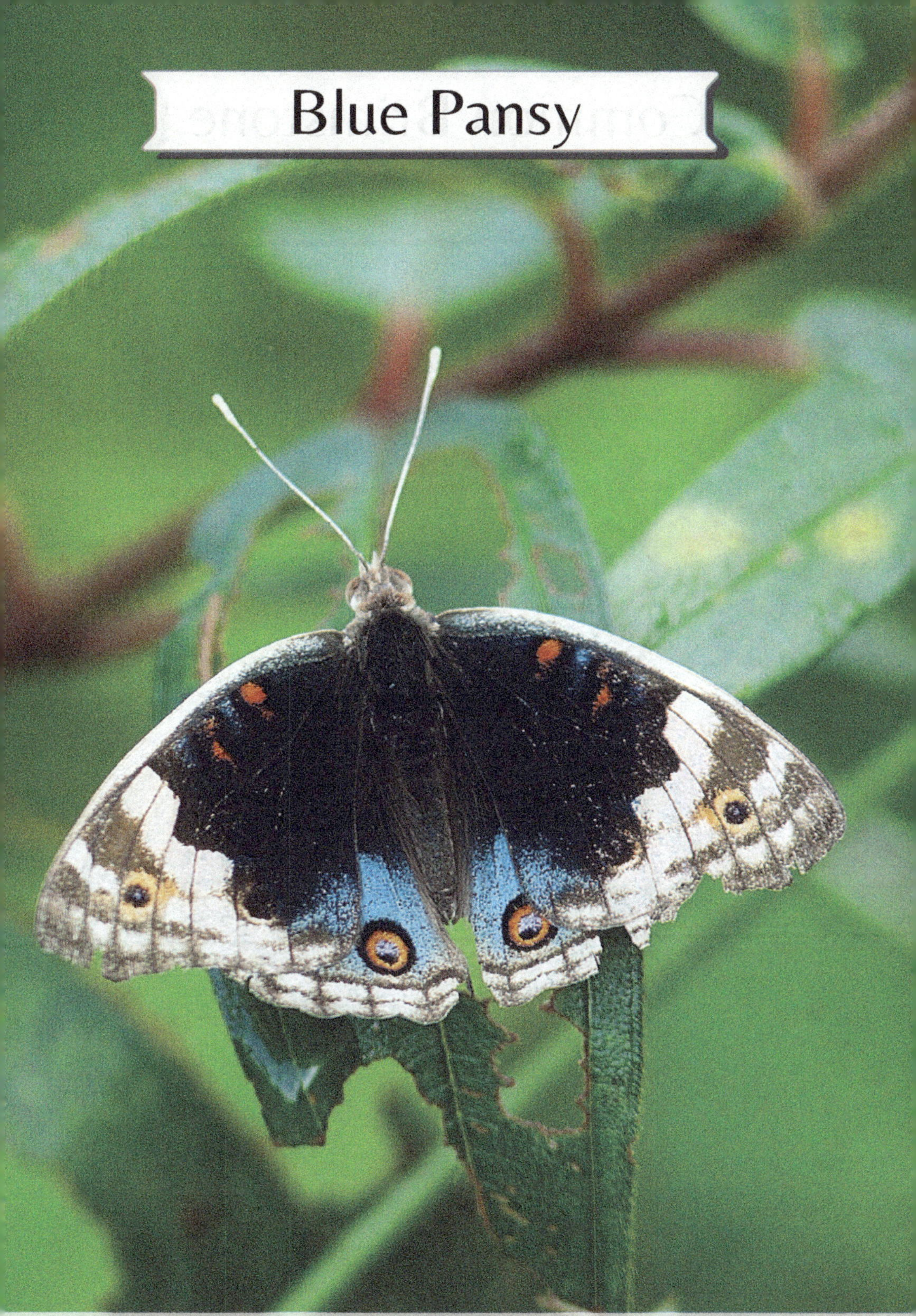

Notice the striking eyespots on bright blue wings.

Common Brimstone

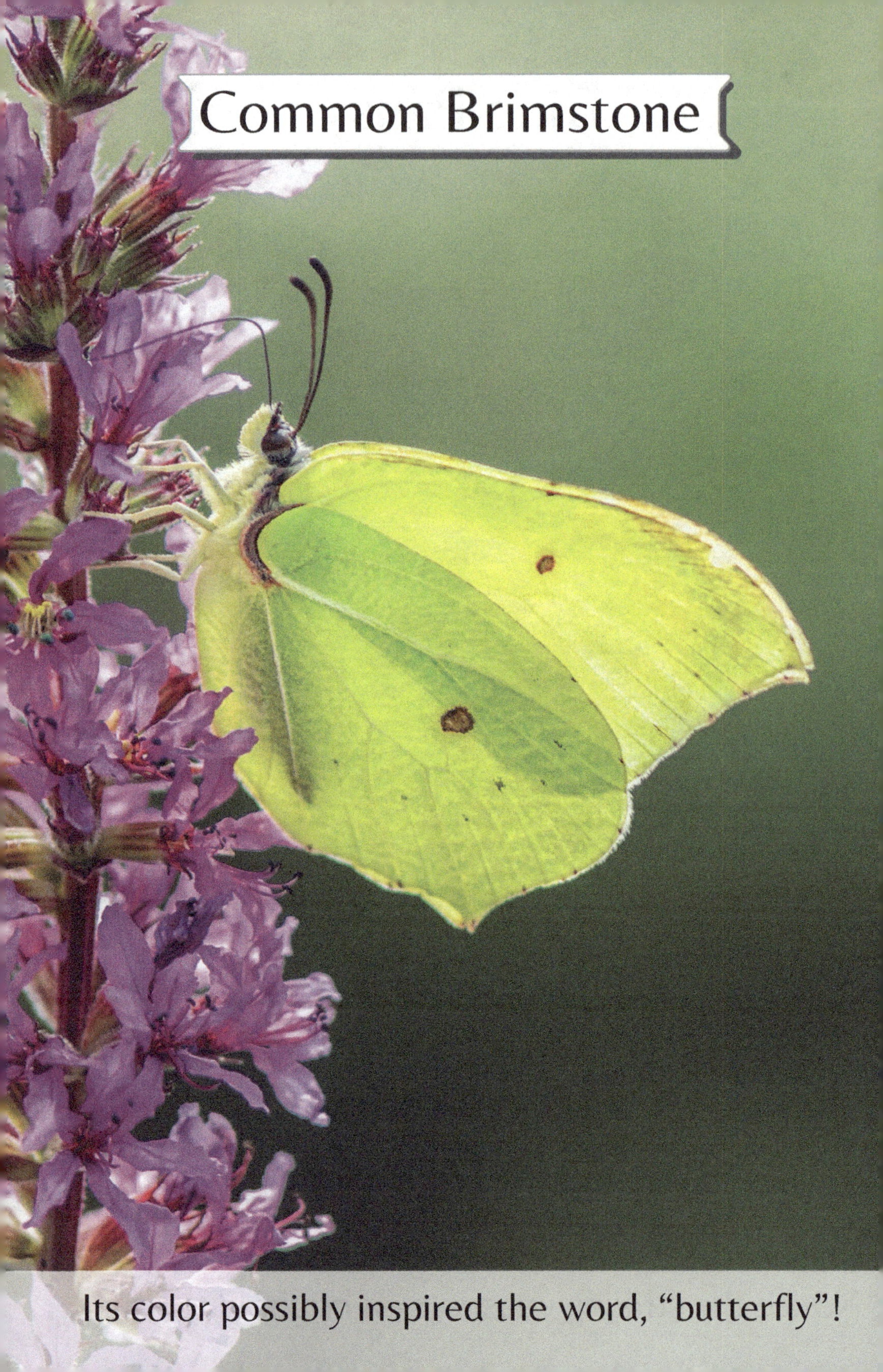

Its color possibly inspired the word, "butterfly"!

Common Rose

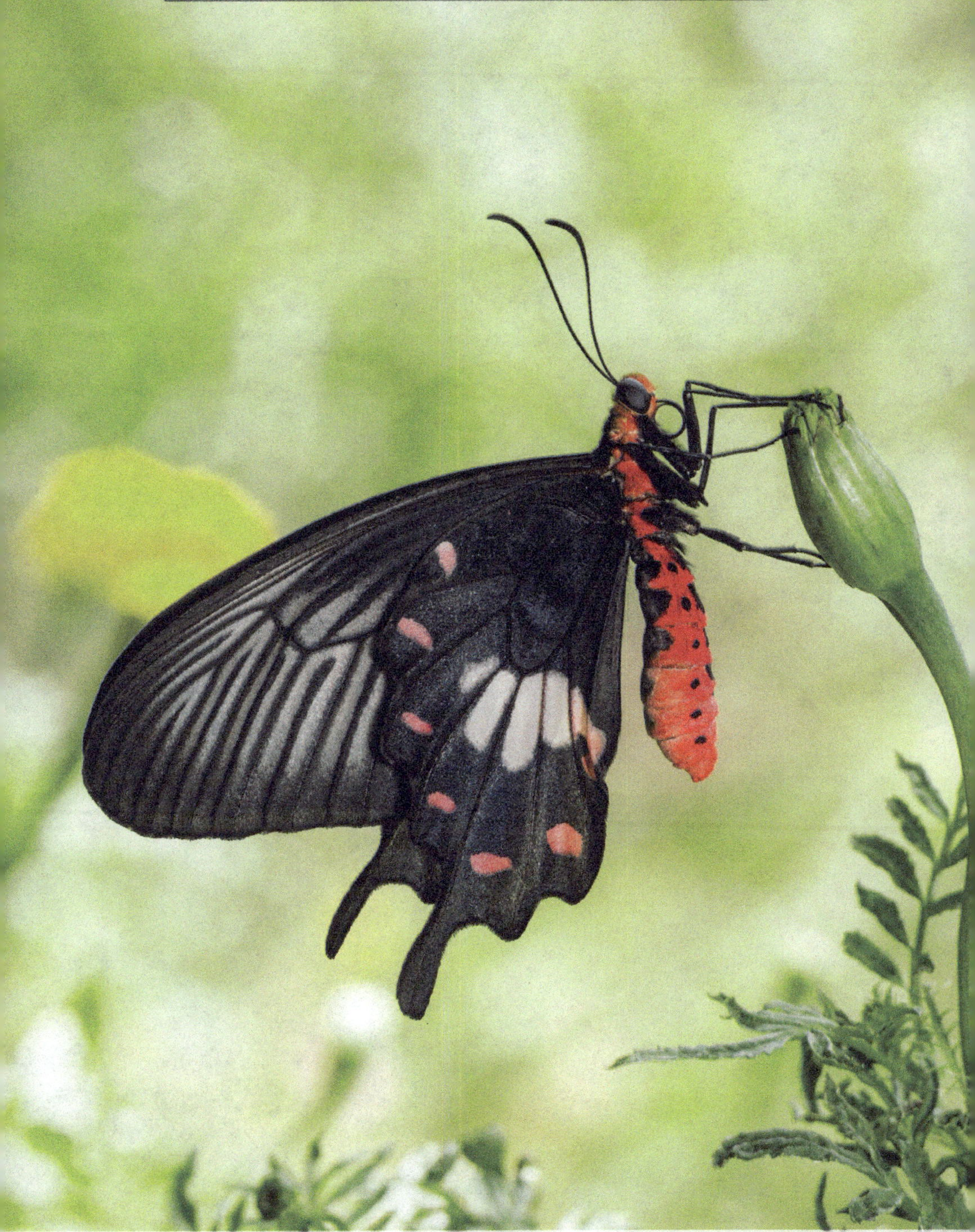

Its colors warn predators that it is toxic!

Lime

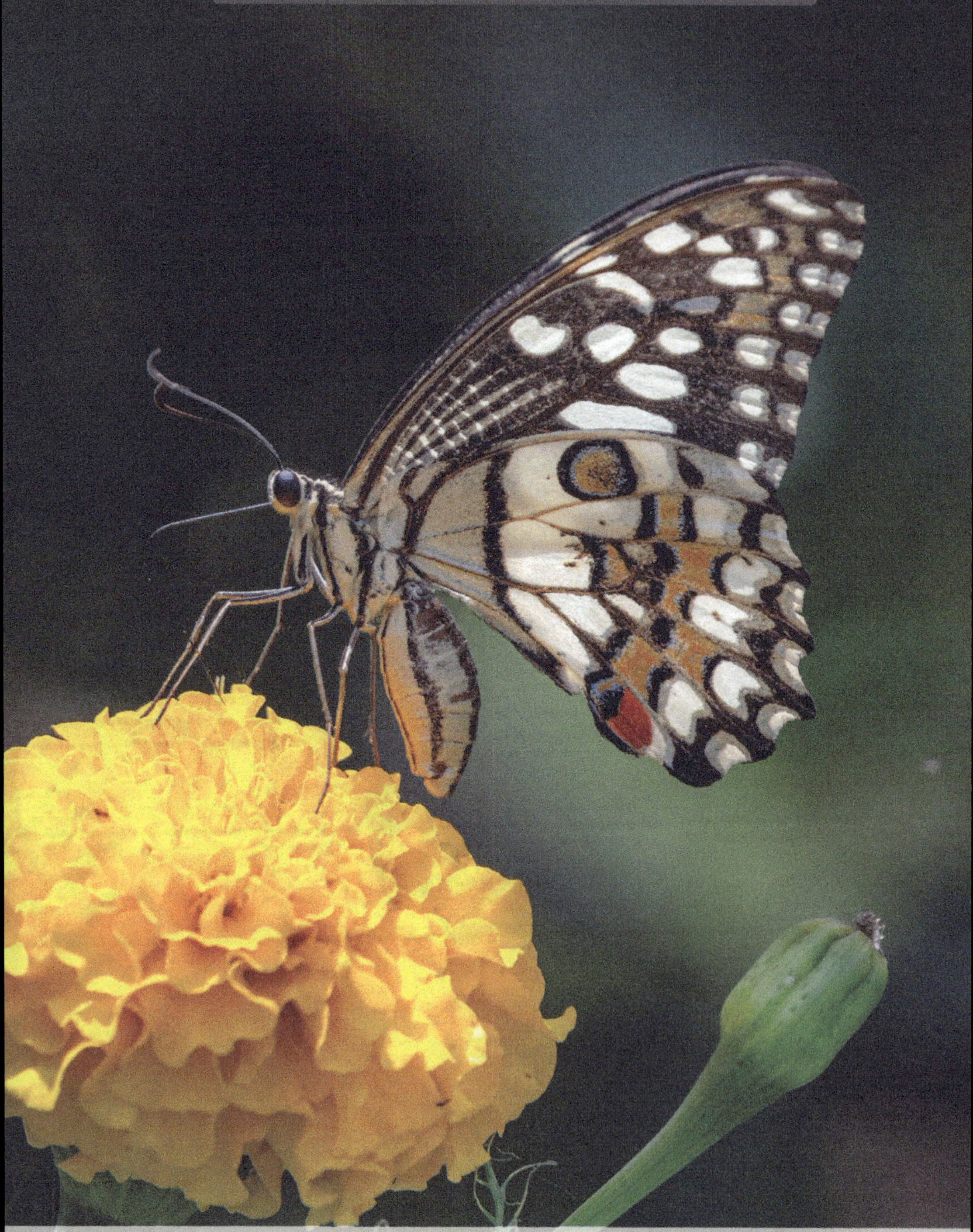

Its caterpillars eat citrus trees before becoming butterflies.

Birdwing

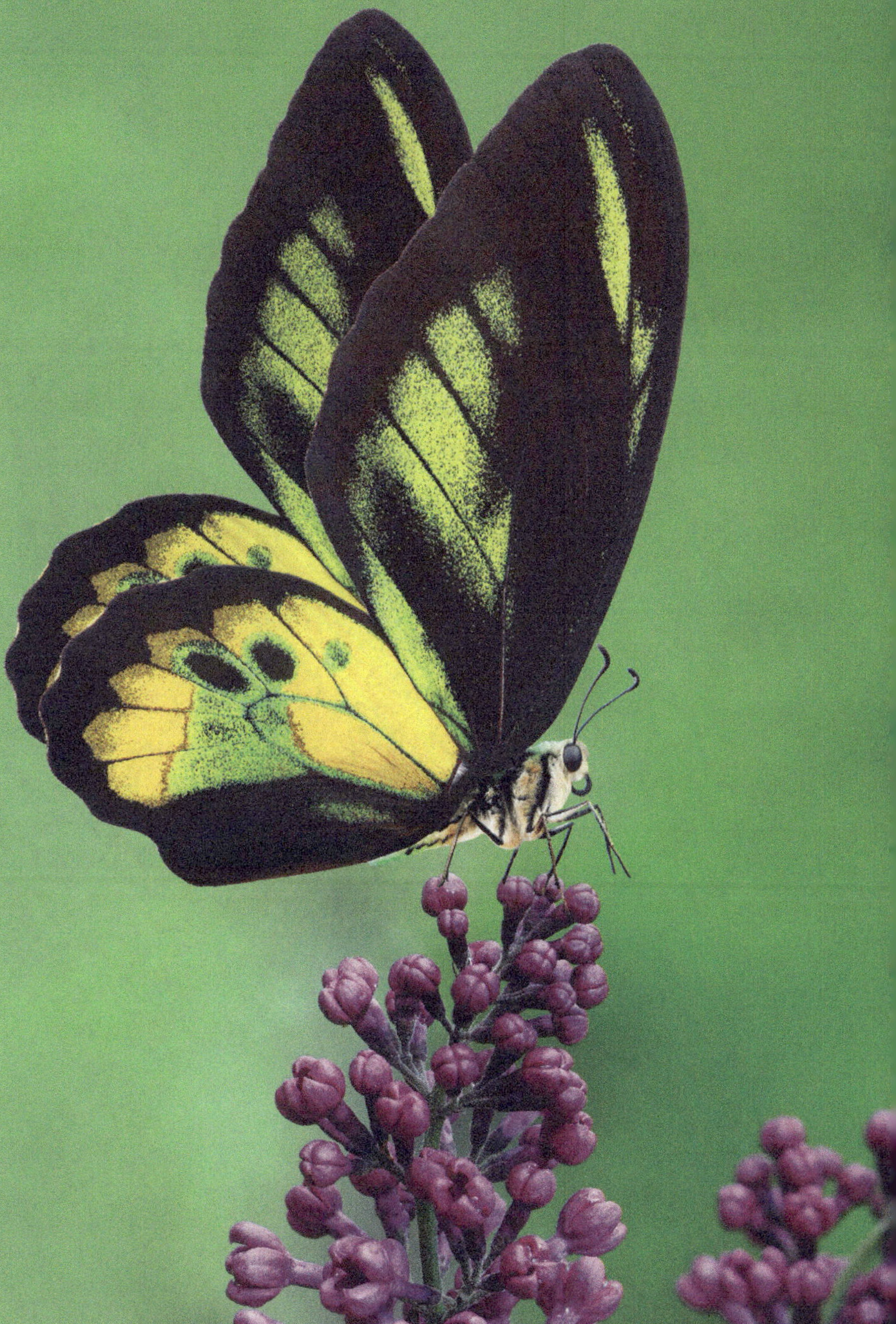

Some grow up to 12 inches wide!

Old World Swallowtail

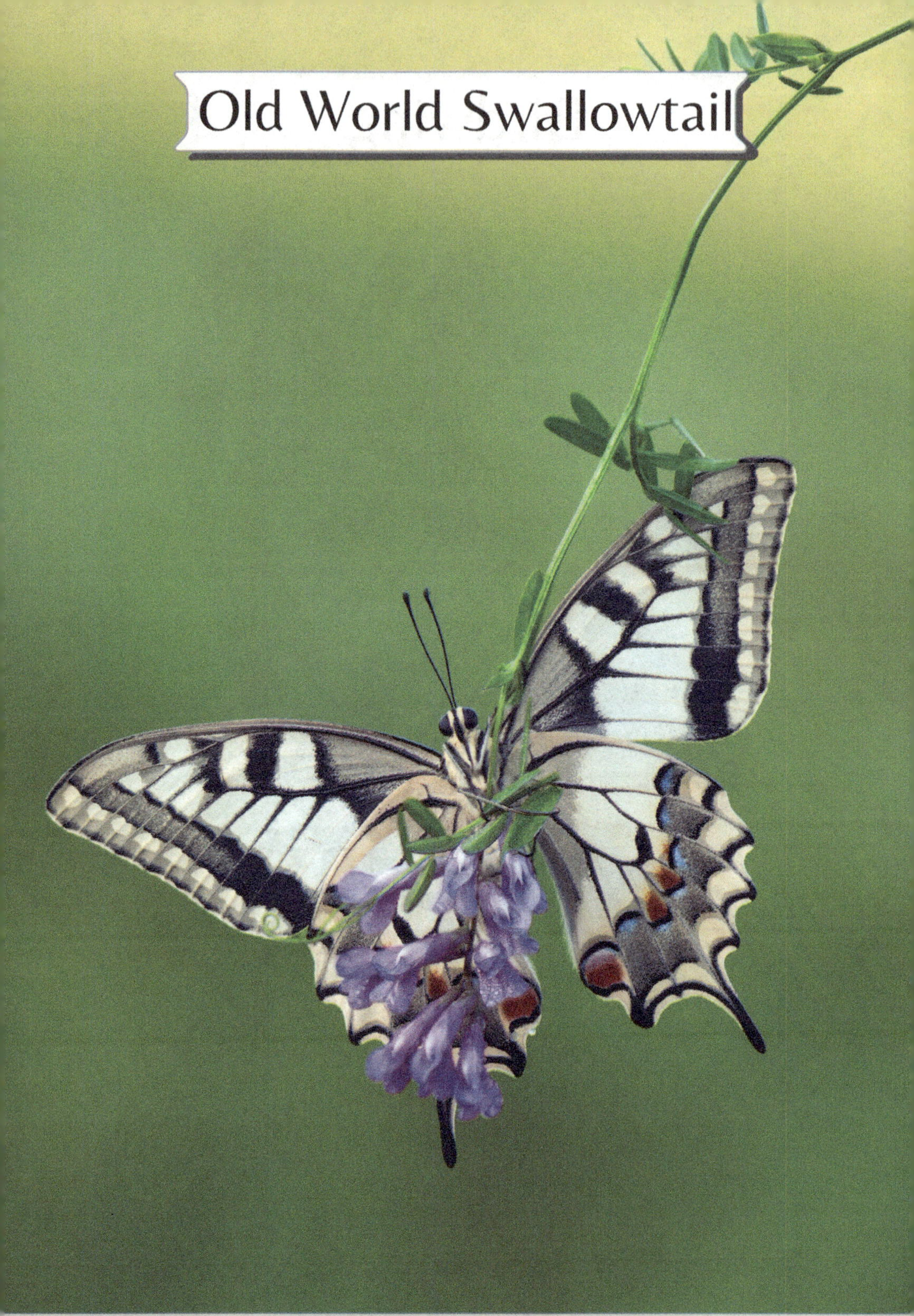

A large butterfly, found across Europe and Asia.

Black-veined White

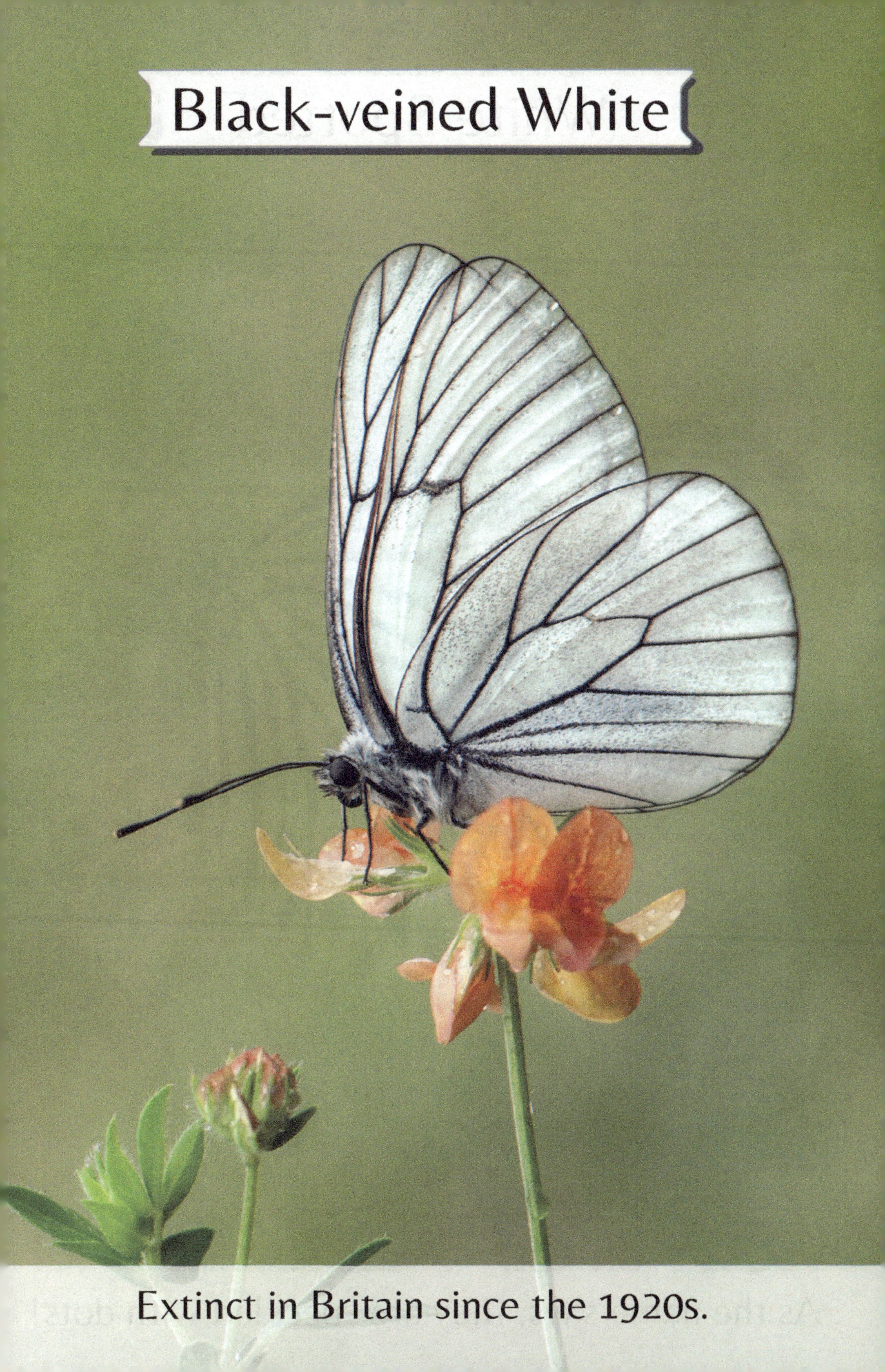

Extinct in Britain since the 1920s.

White Spotted

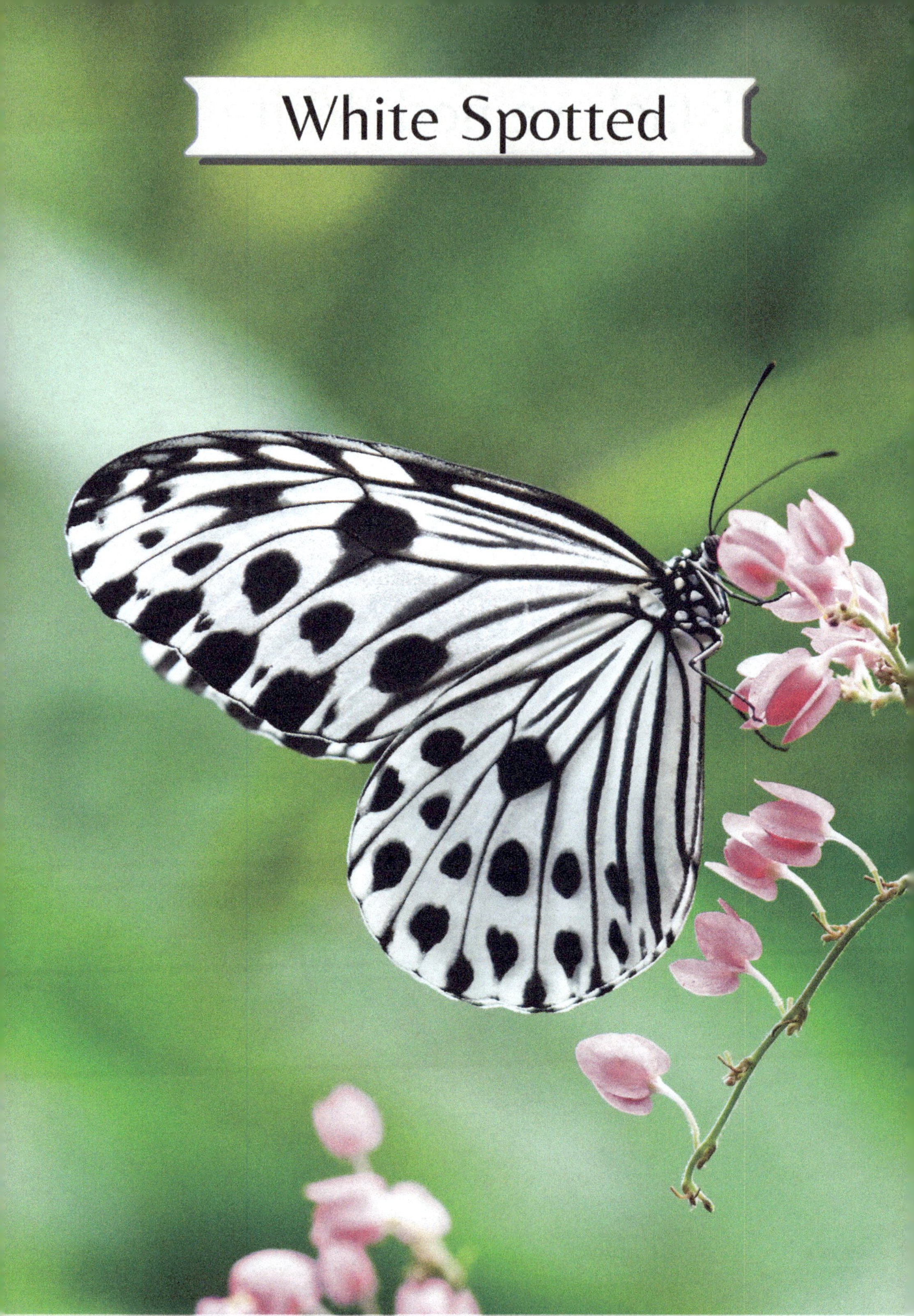

As the name says, they are speckled with dots!

Marbled White

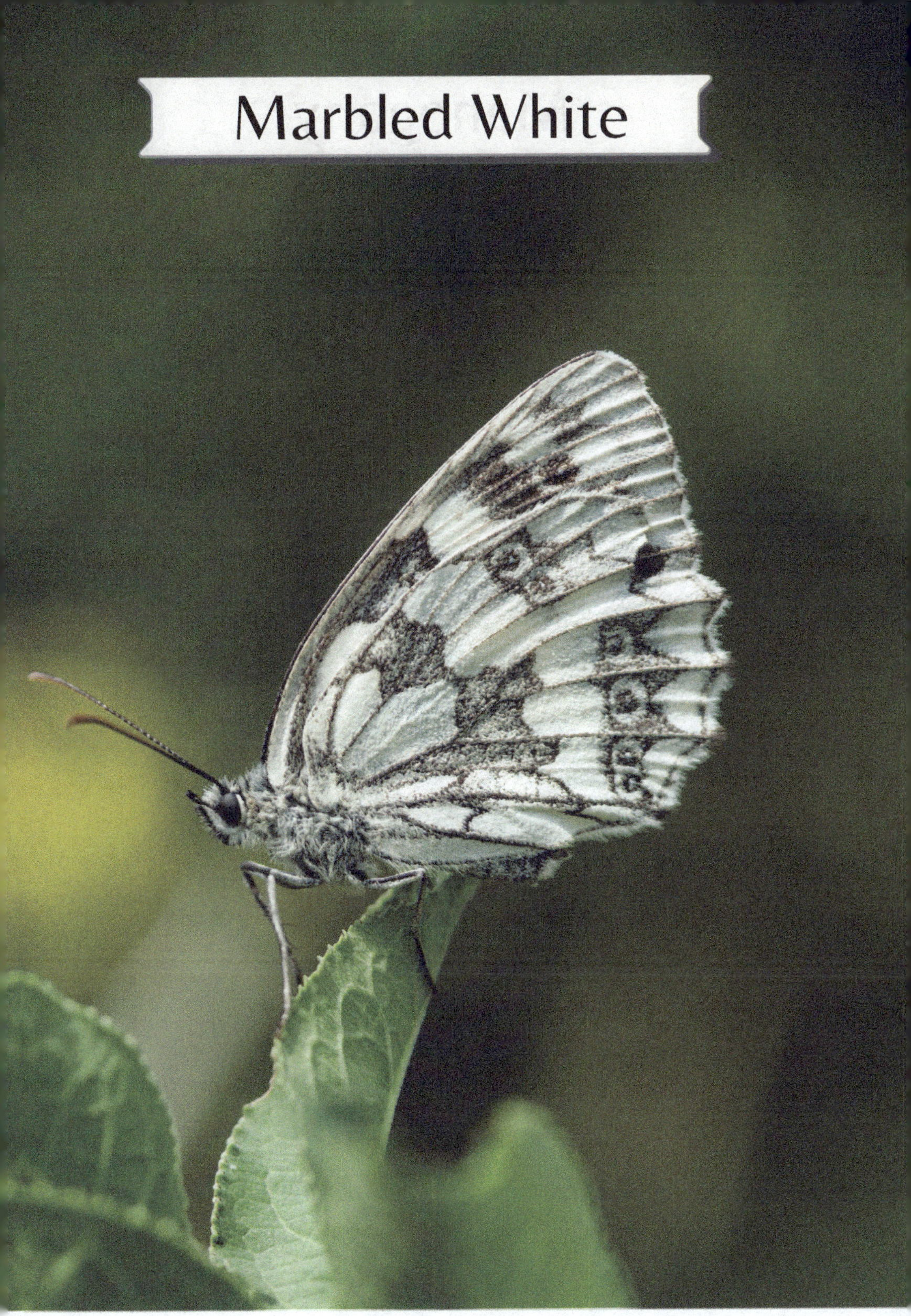

They have striking checkerboard looking wings!

Mahogany

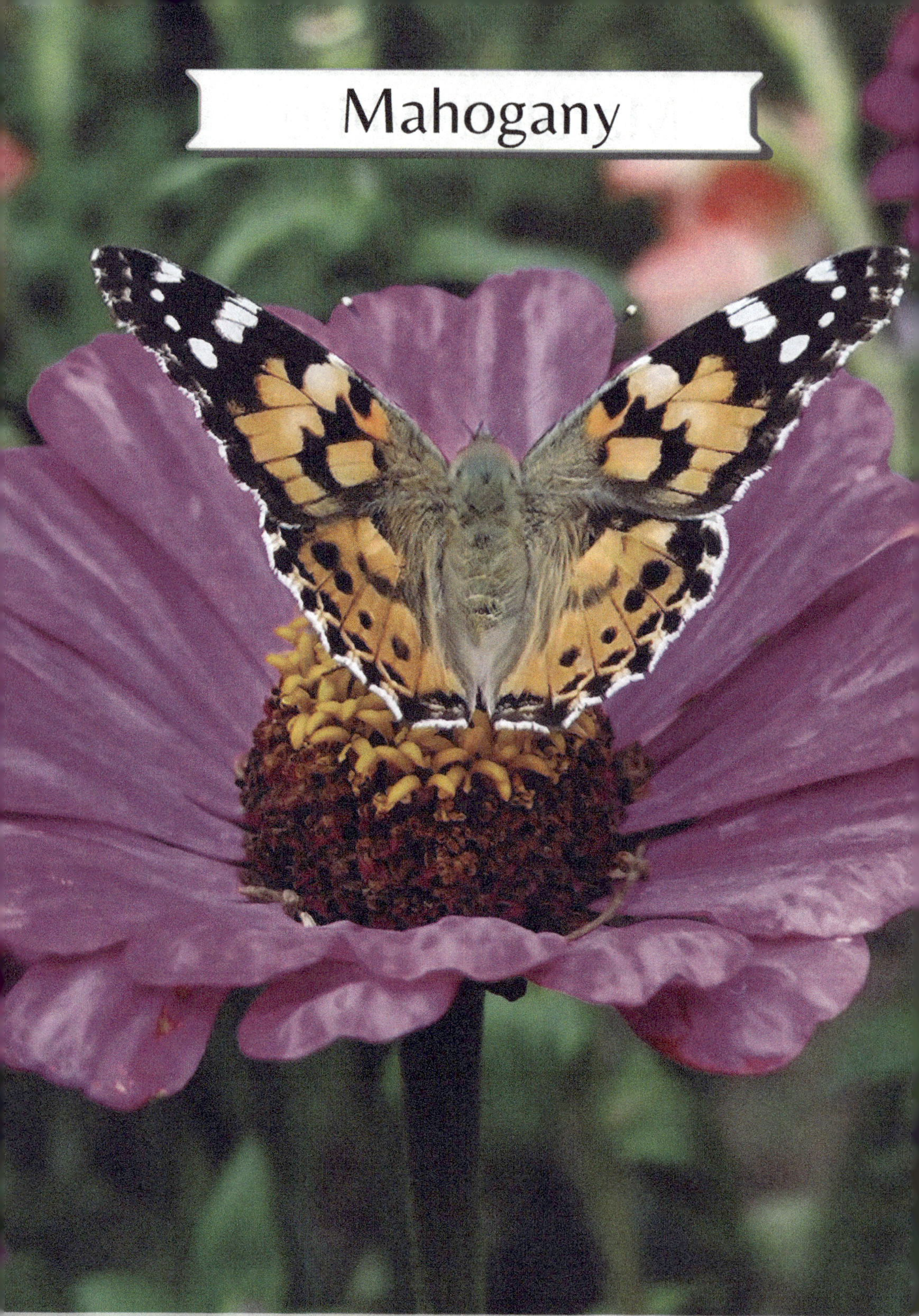

Their rich brown wings look like polished wood.

Blue Morpho

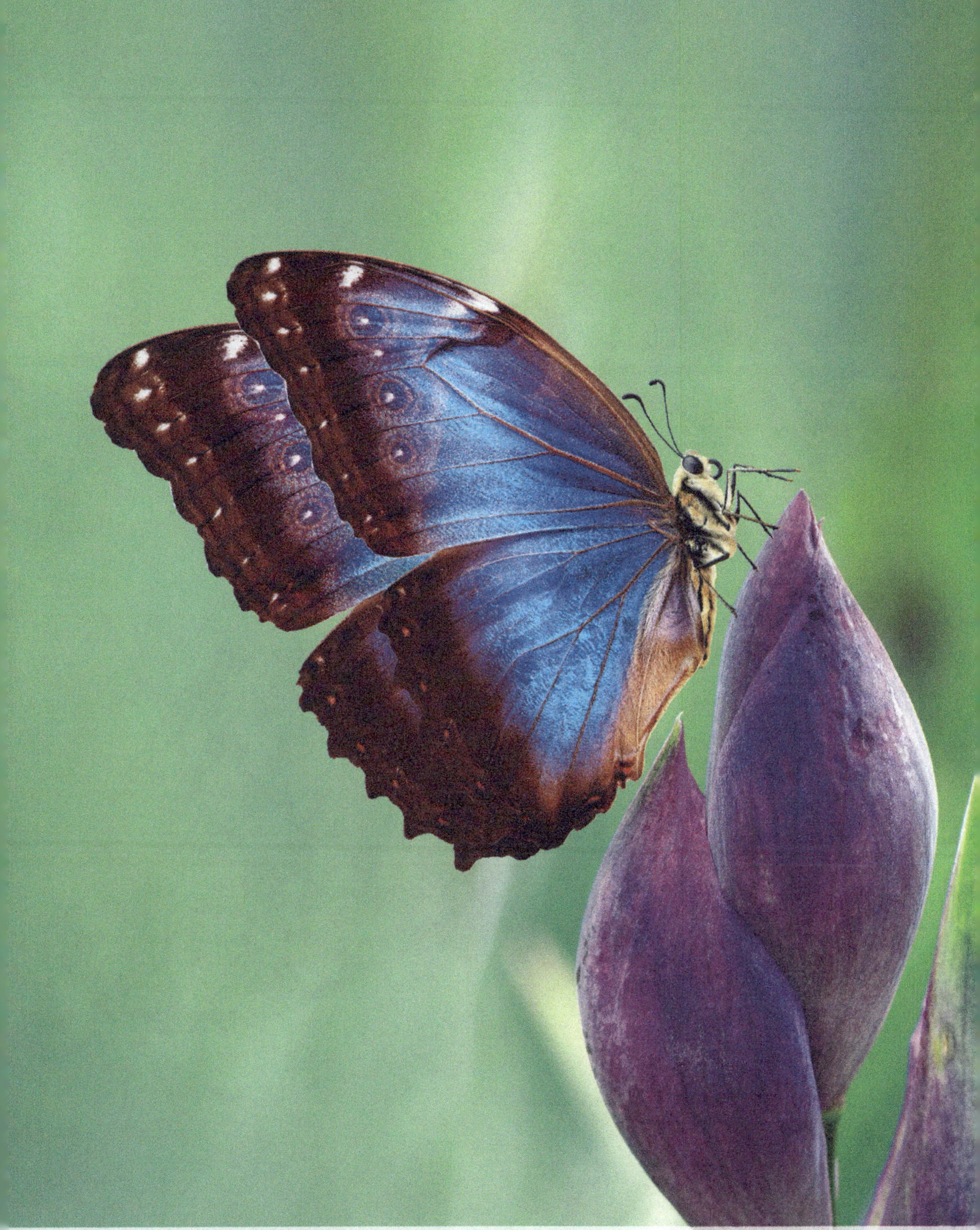

Their blue wings dazzle when they're flying!

Tawny Coaster

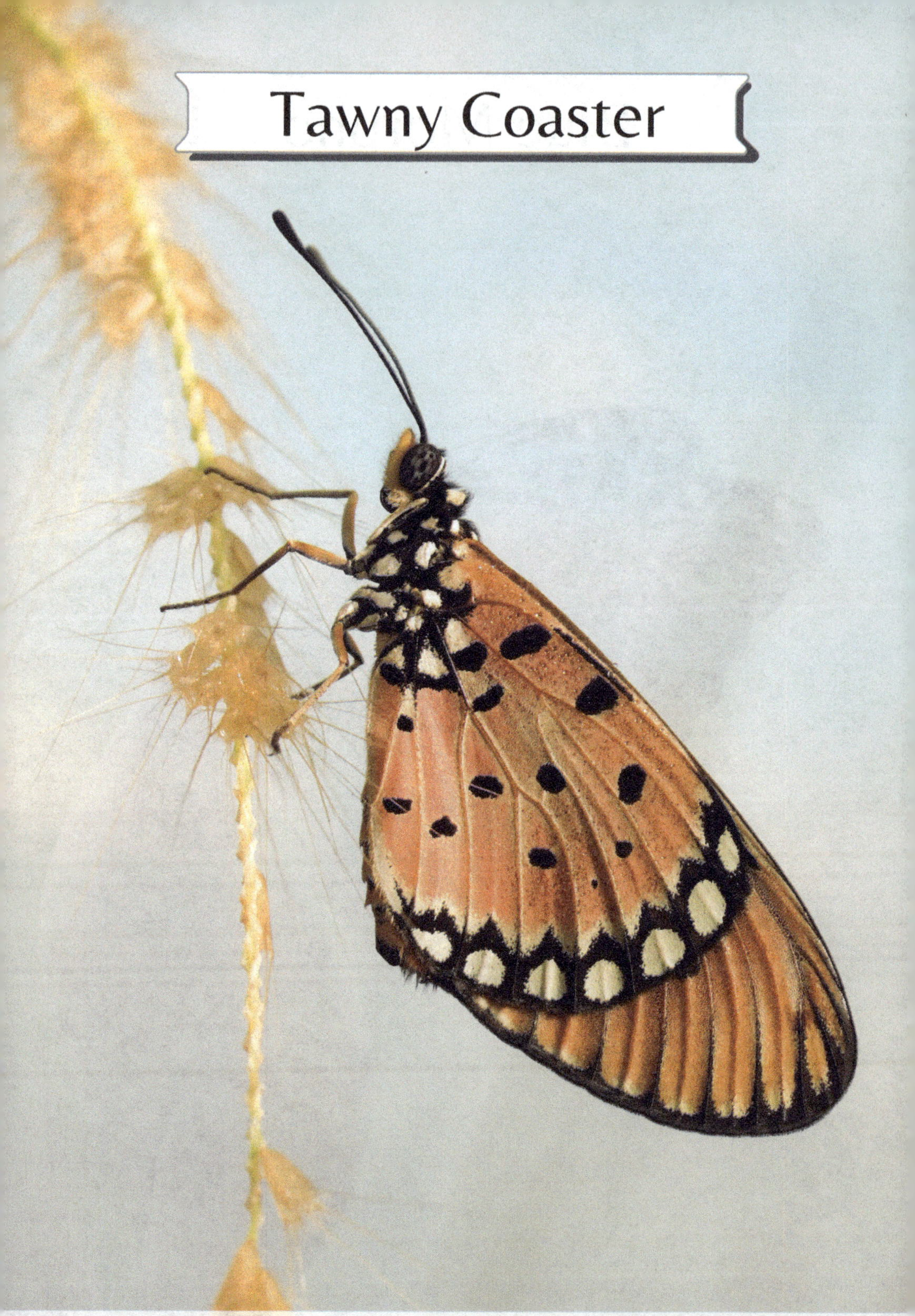

Native to India & Sri Lanka, now expanding across Asia.

Blue Moon

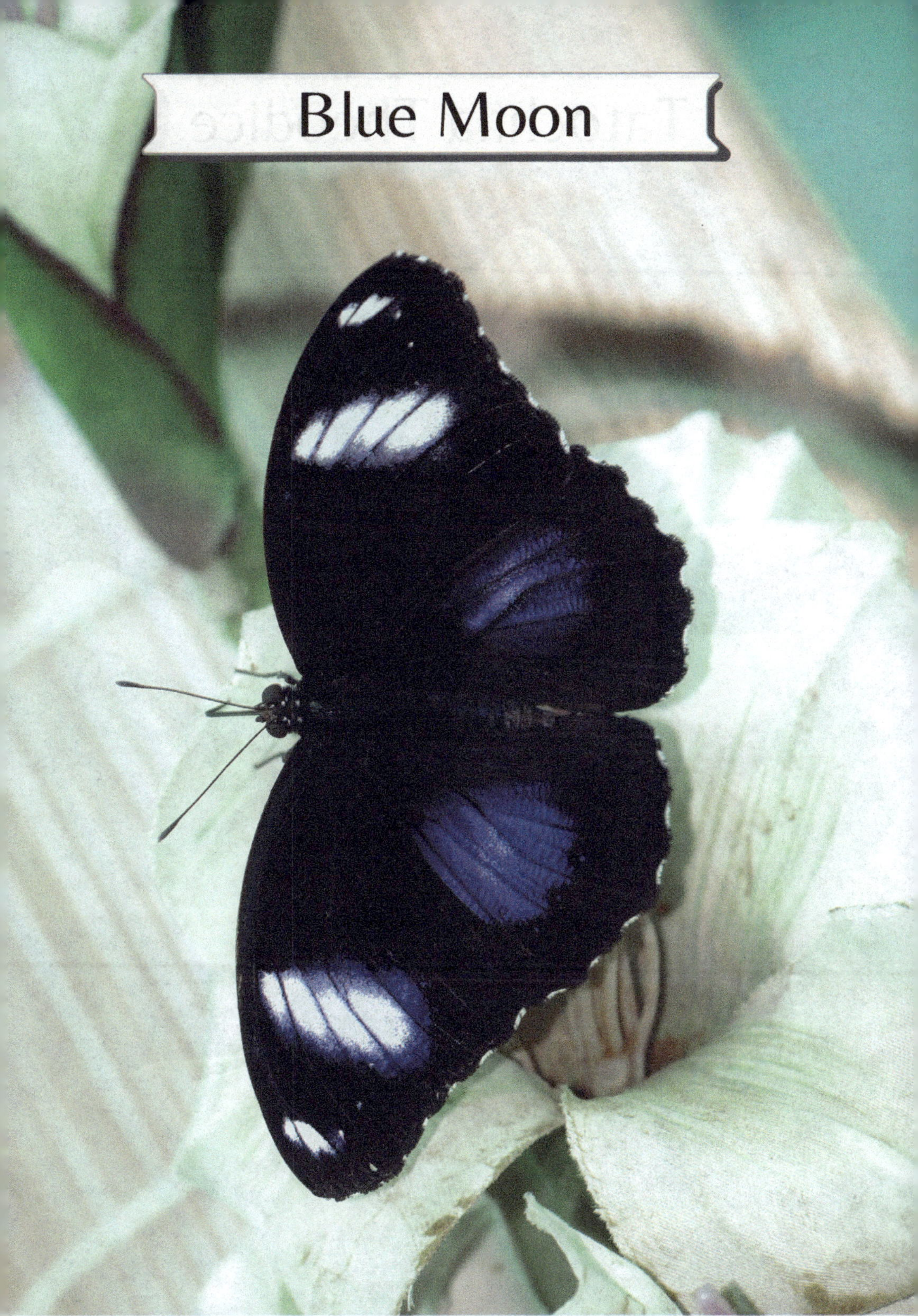

The females mimic toxic butterfly species' looks!

Tatochila Theodice

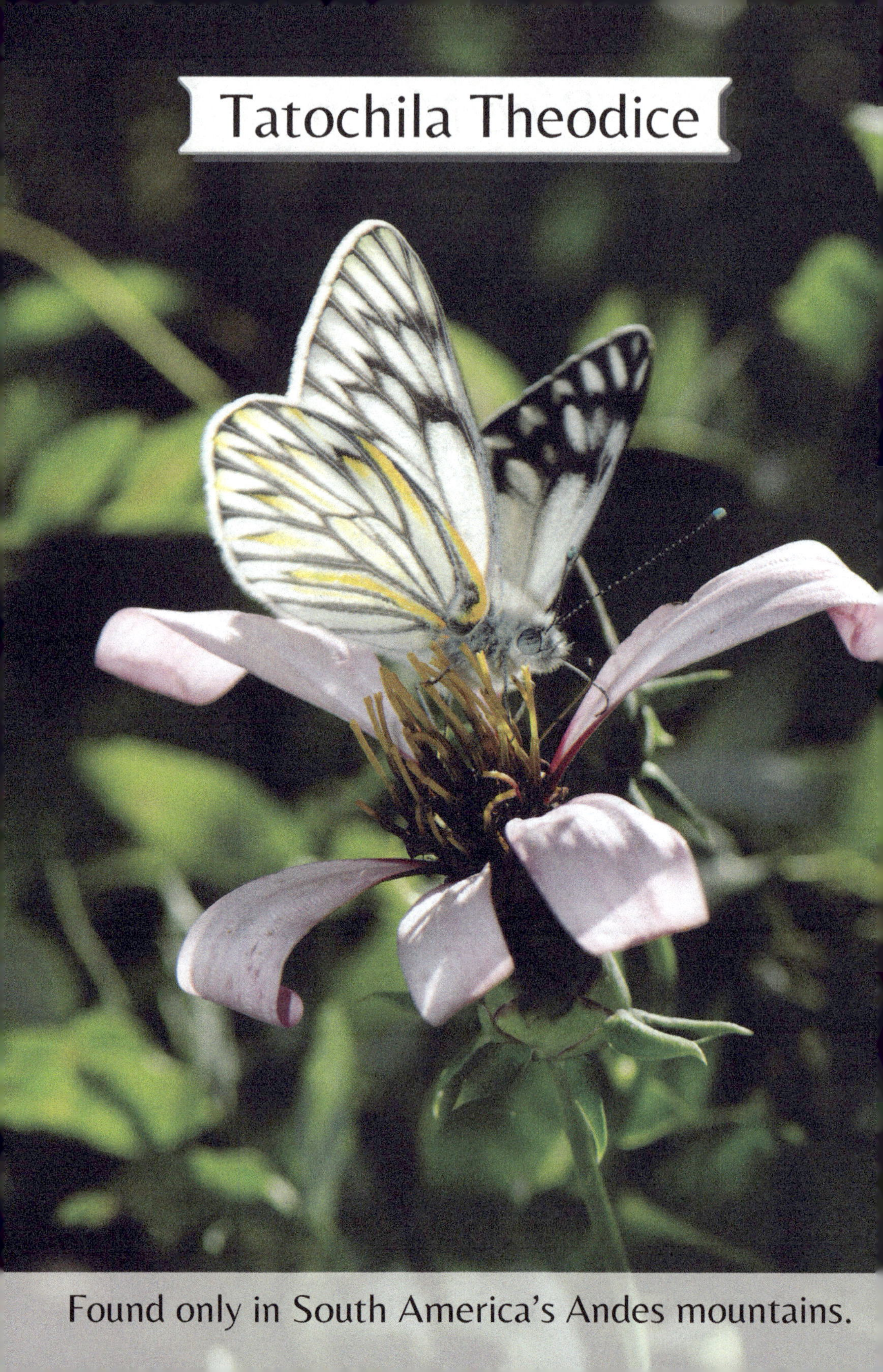

Found only in South America's Andes mountains.

Lesser Fiery Copper

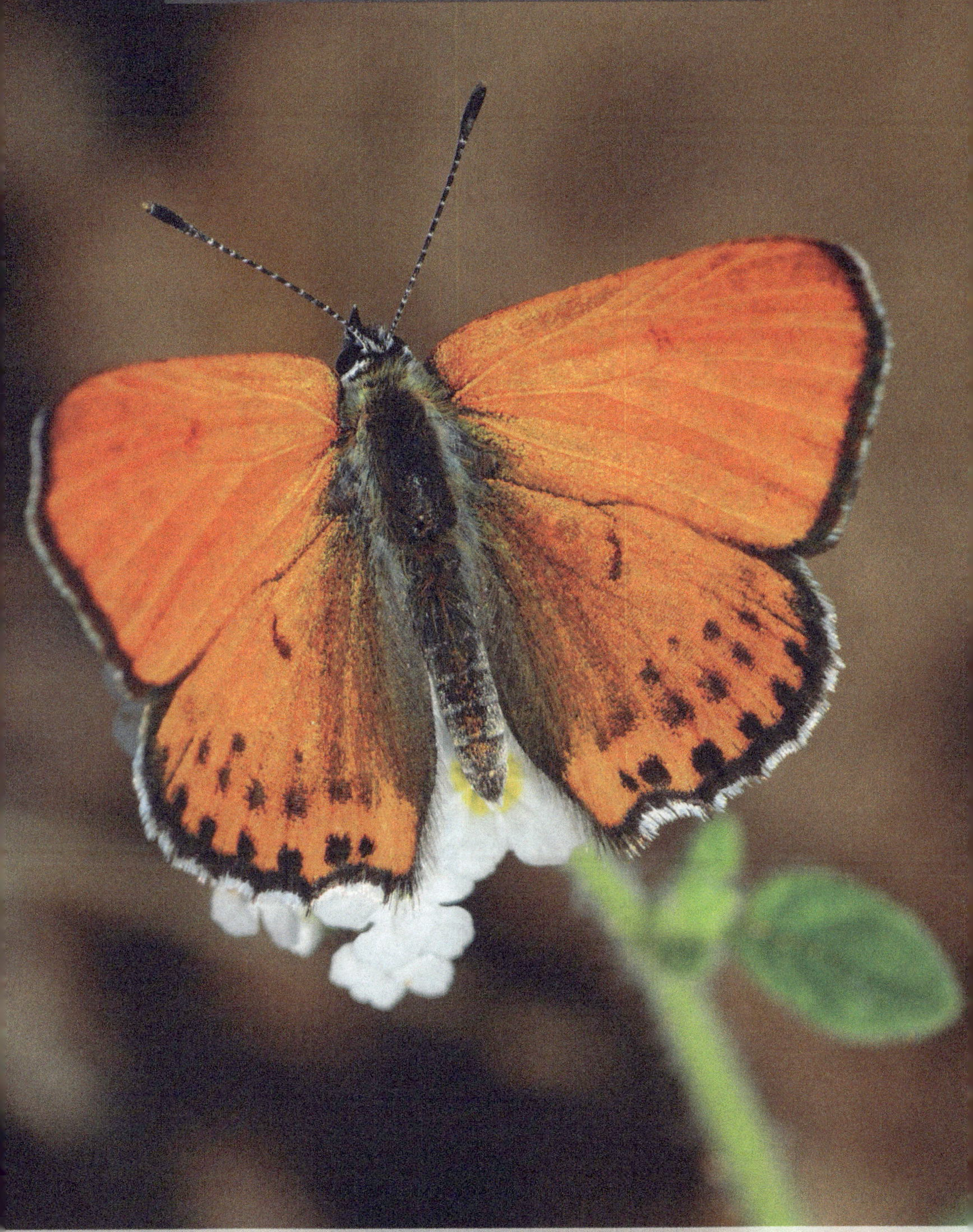

Known for having small "tails" on its hindwings

Red Spotted Purple

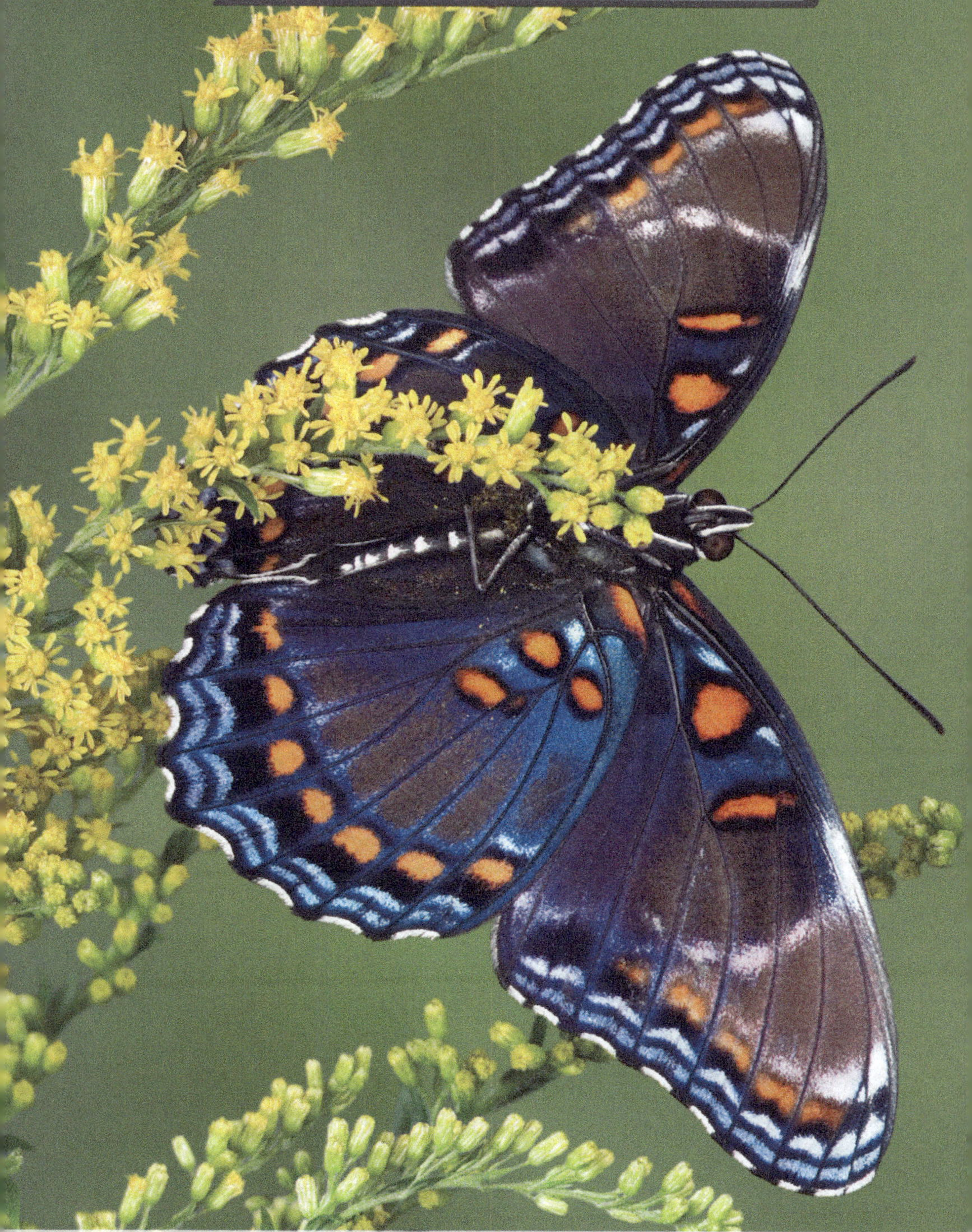

Looks like a Swallowtail butterfly, without the tail!

Great Eggfly

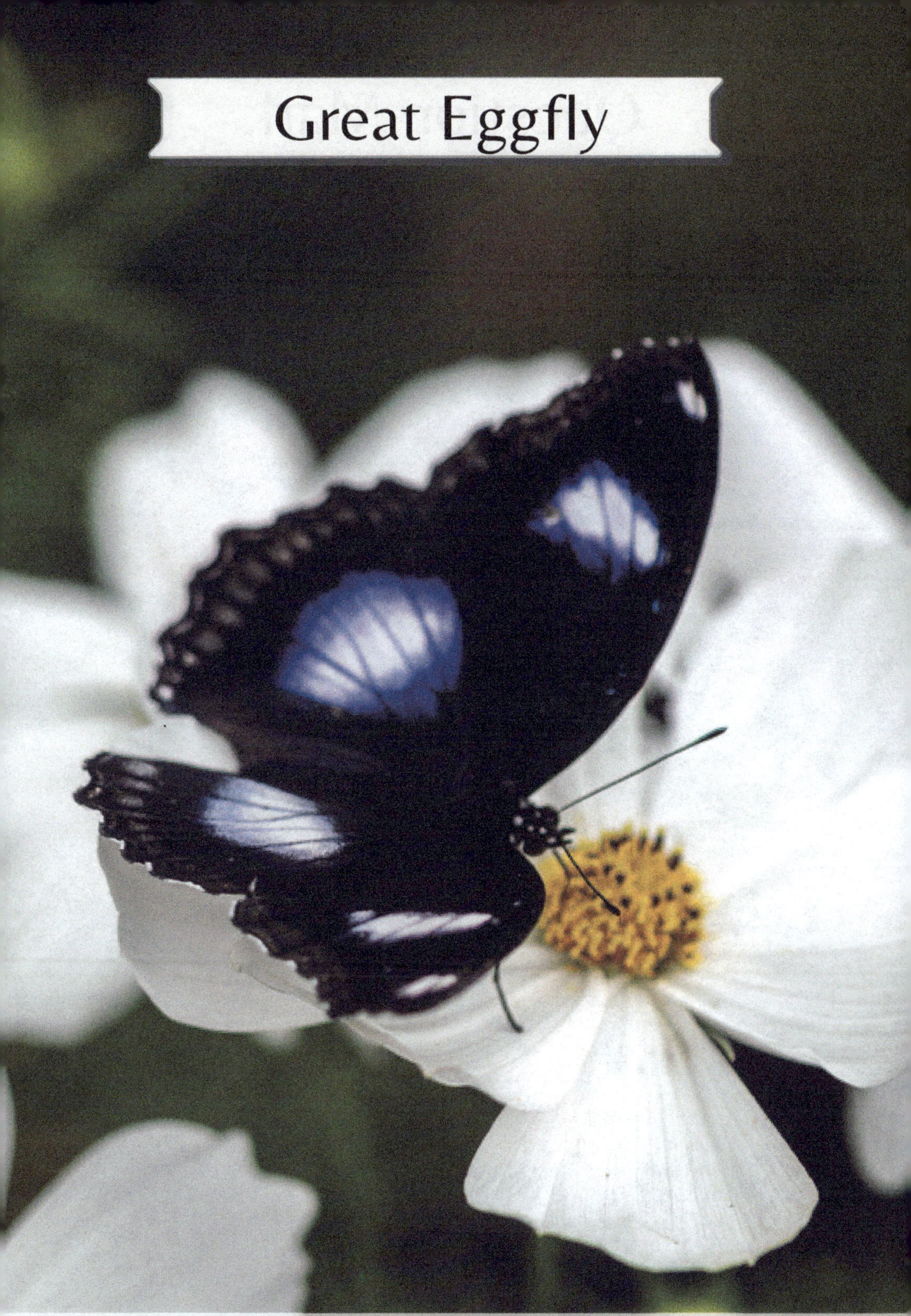

In New Zealand, it is also called the Blue Moon Butterfly.

Question Mark

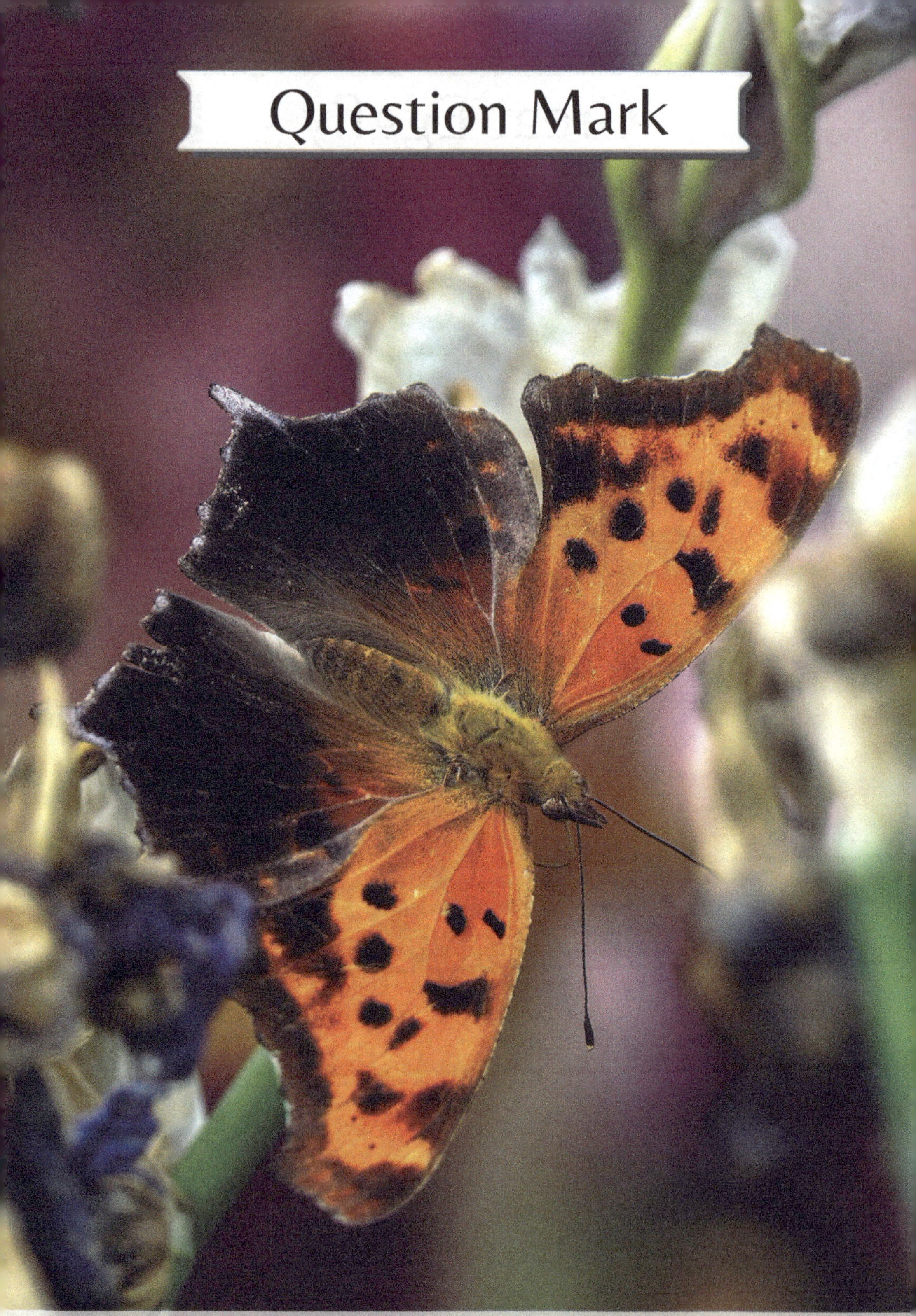

They have a tiny silver "?" mark underneath!

Map

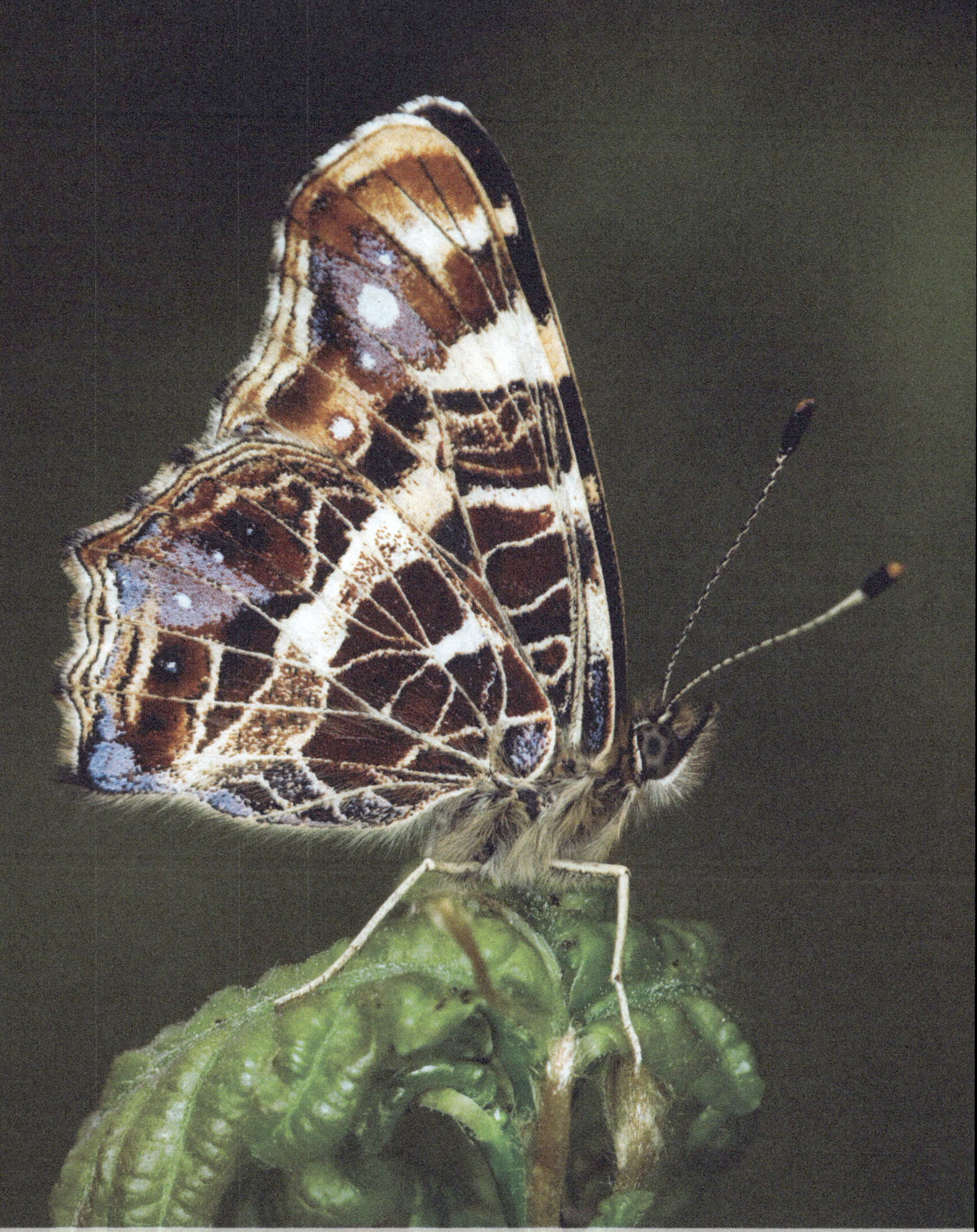

Their wing veins resemble a road map!

Scarce Swallowtail

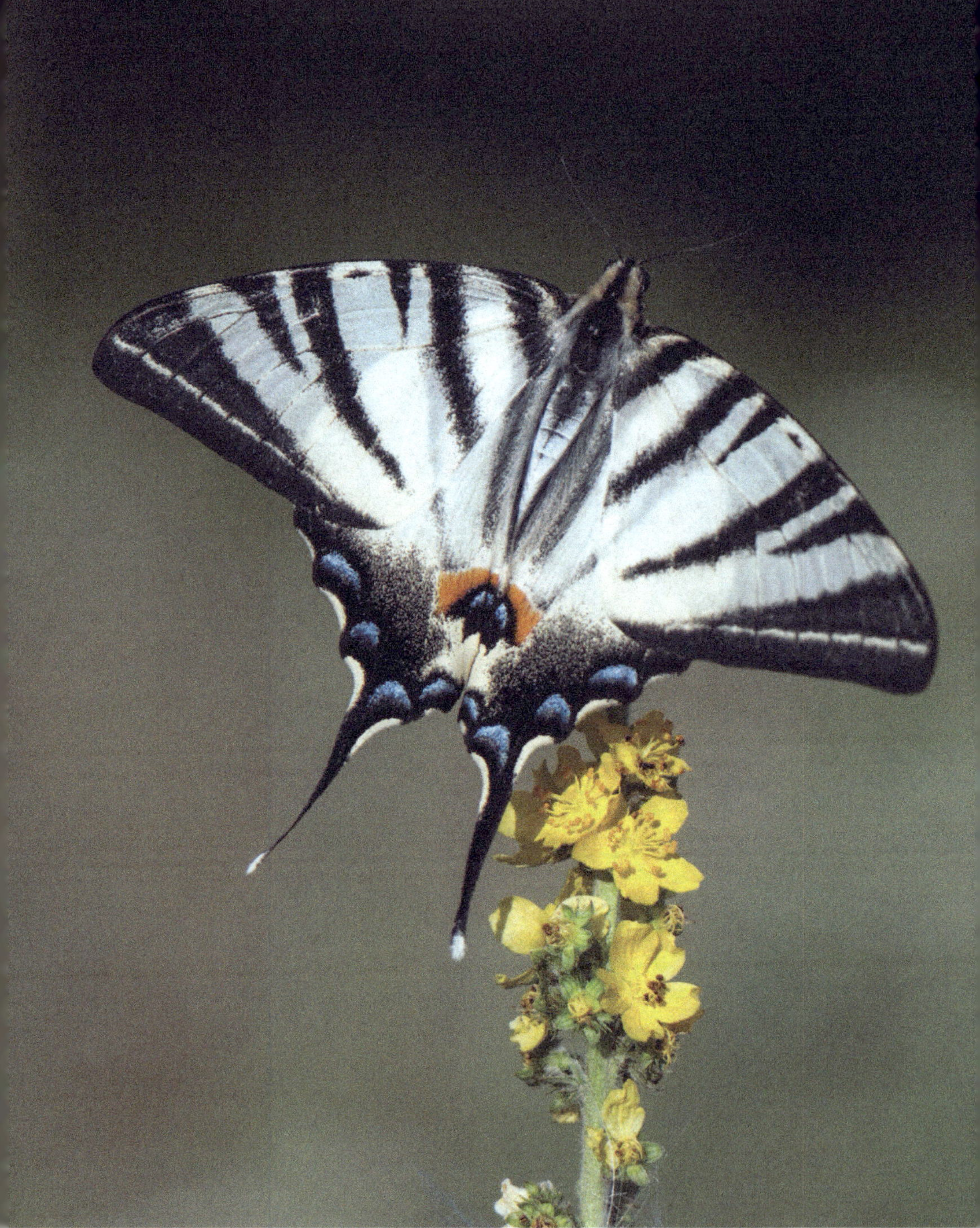

Despite their name, they are actually quite common!

Small Postman

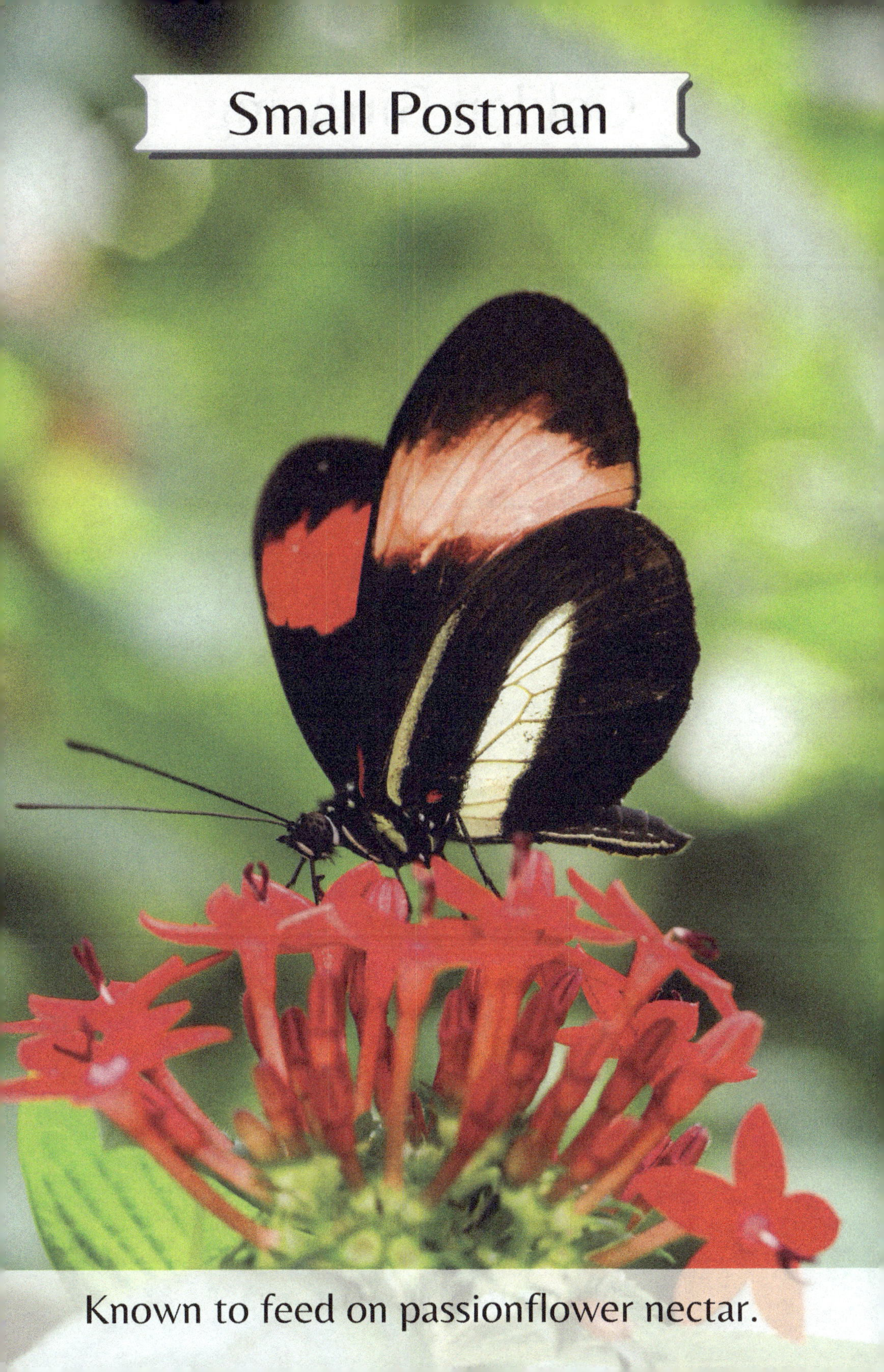

Known to feed on passionflower nectar.

Golden Birdwing

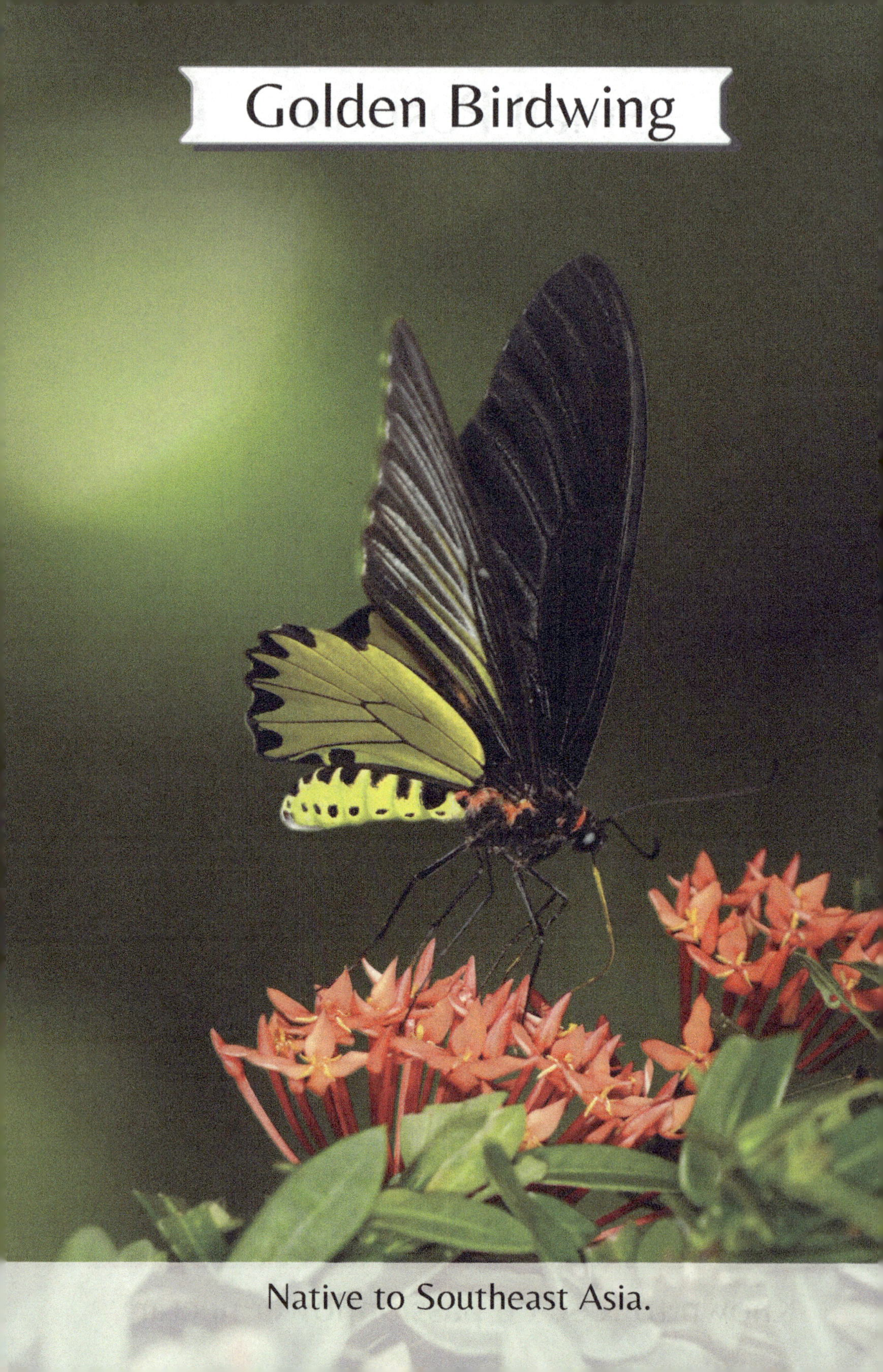

Native to Southeast Asia.

Tiger Longwing

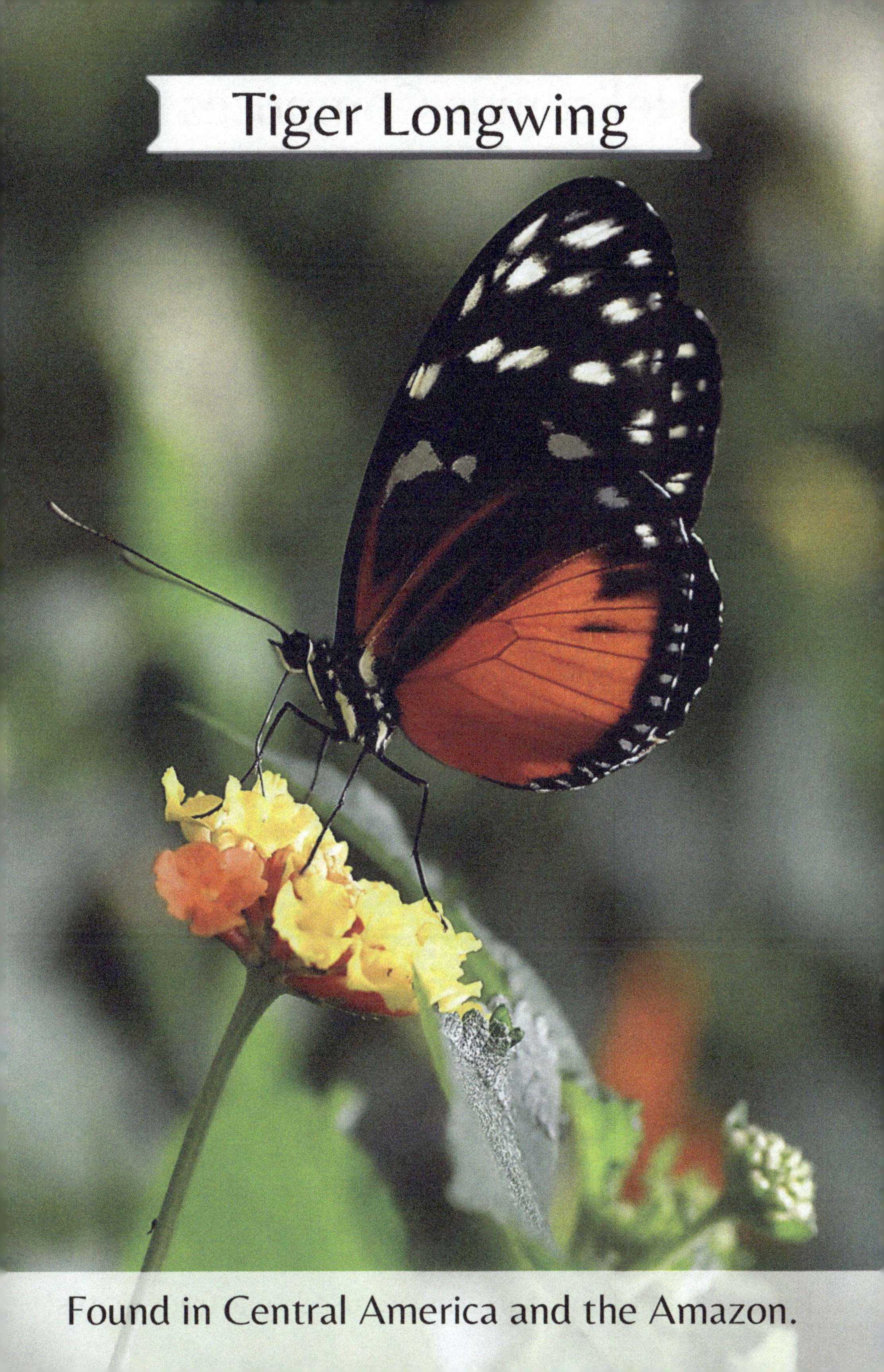

Found in Central America and the Amazon.

Heliconius Comprises

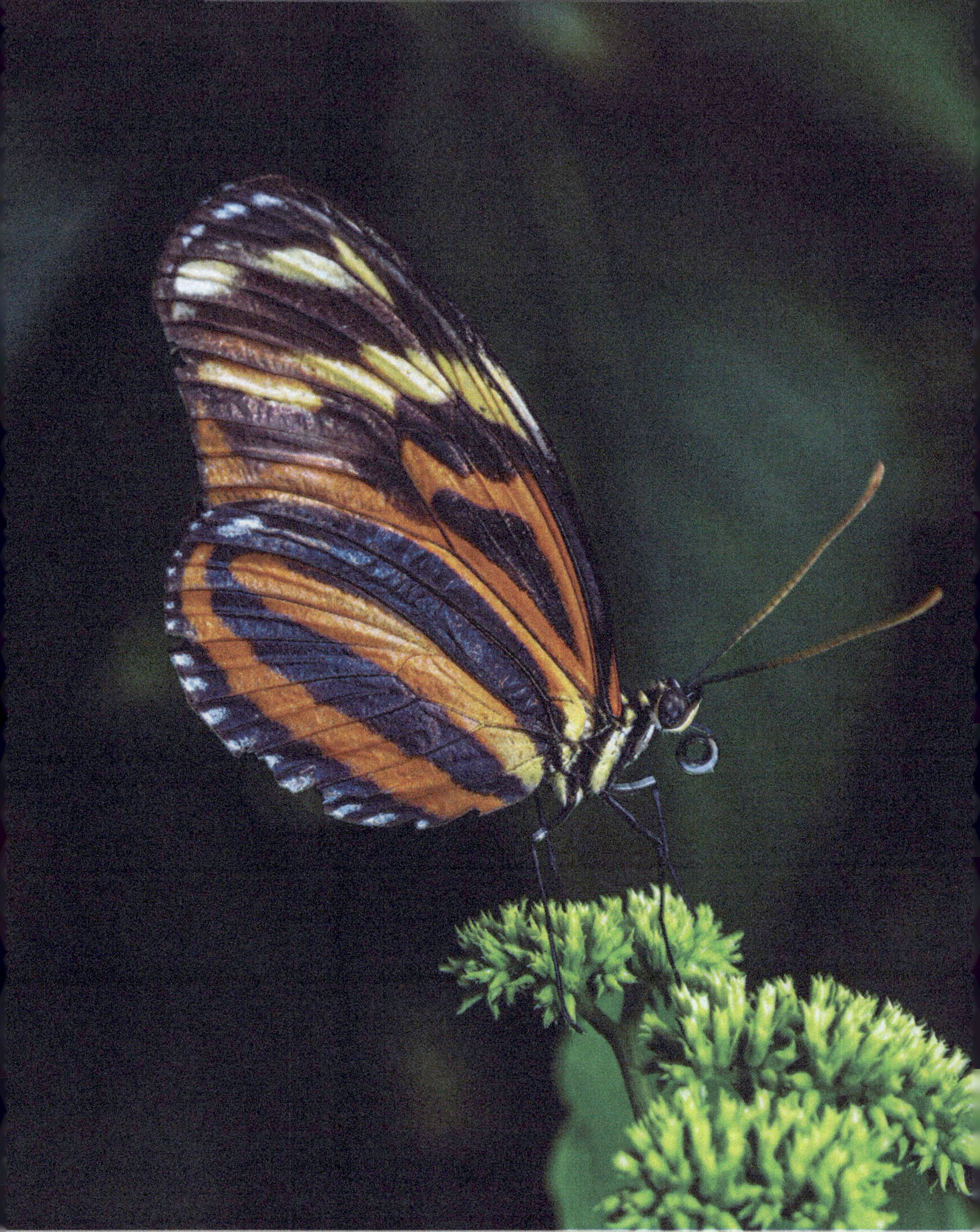

Their striking wing patterns are used to attract mates!

Common Jezebel

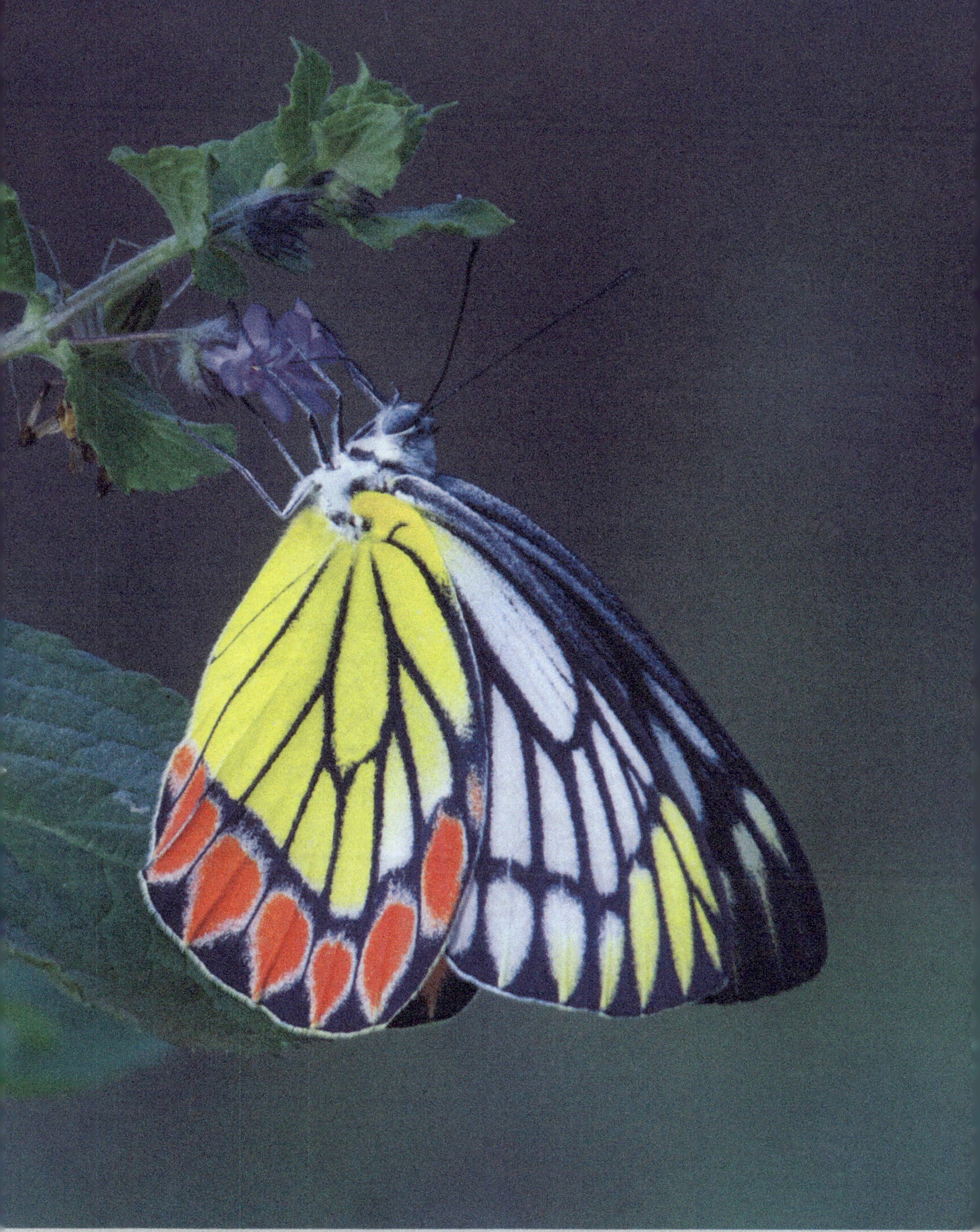

Their bright colors warn birds they taste bad!

King Swallowtail

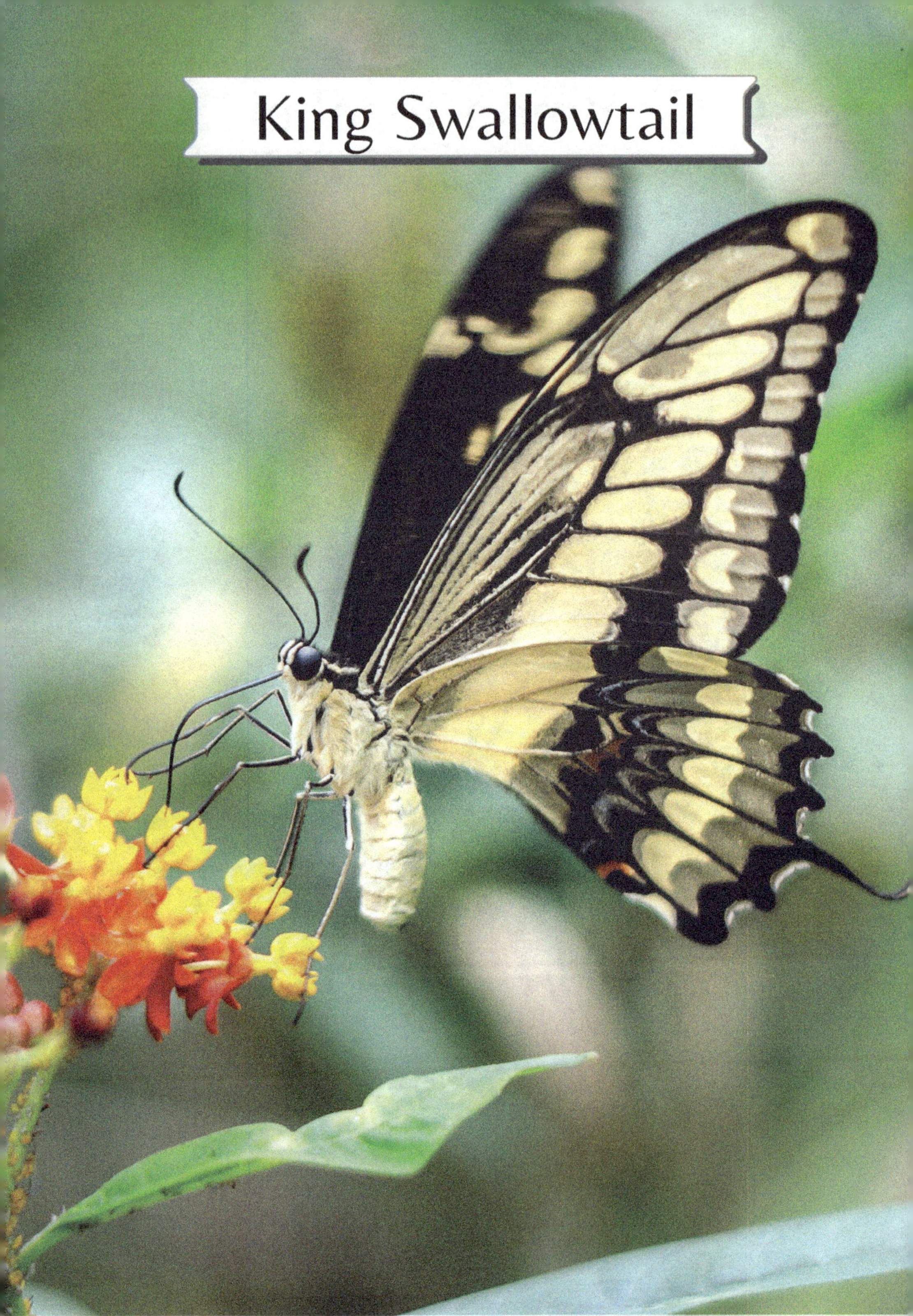

One of the world's largest butterflies!

Tailed Jay

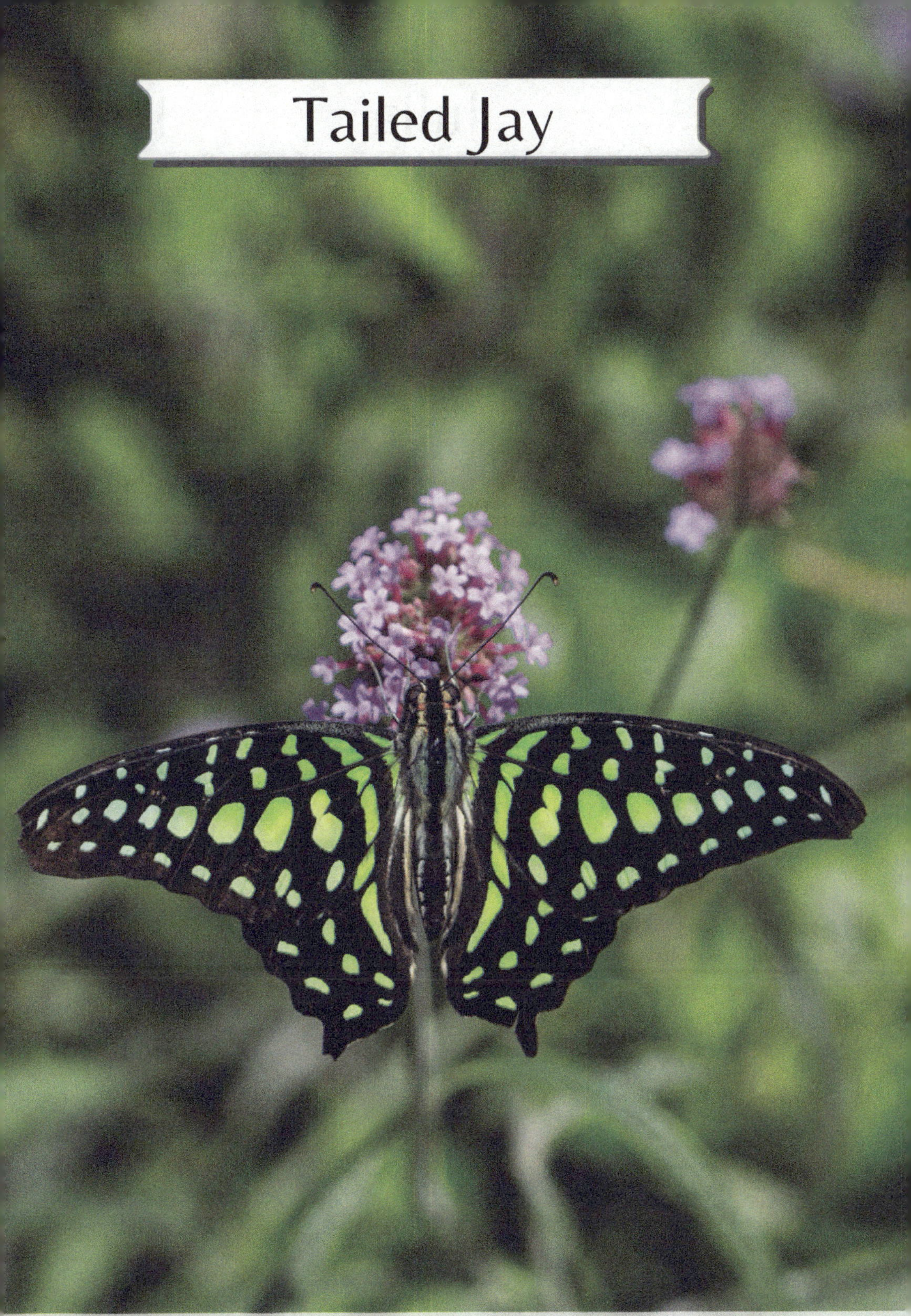

A unique species native to Southeast Asia.

Julia

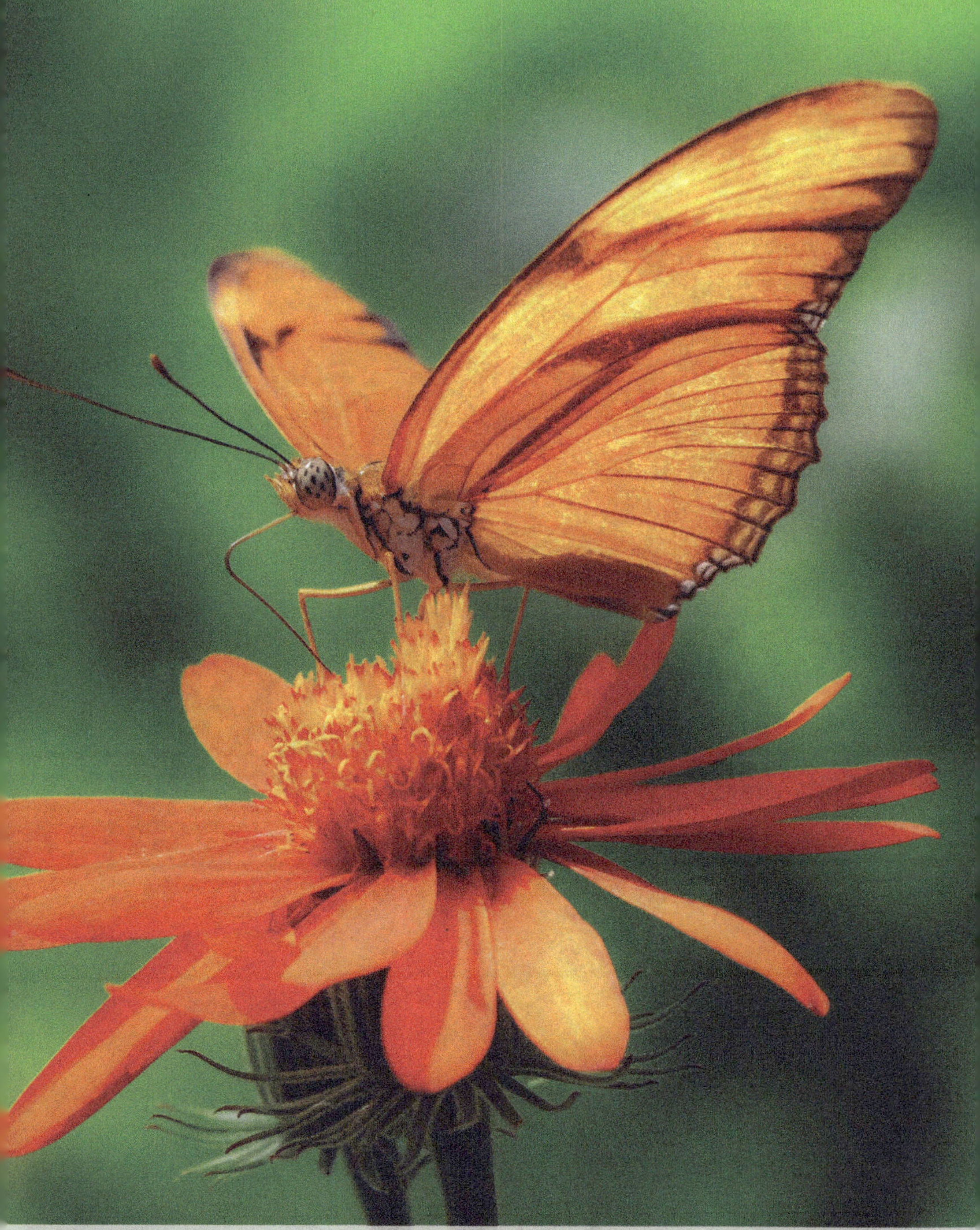

They make turtles cry to drink their tears!

Plain Tiger

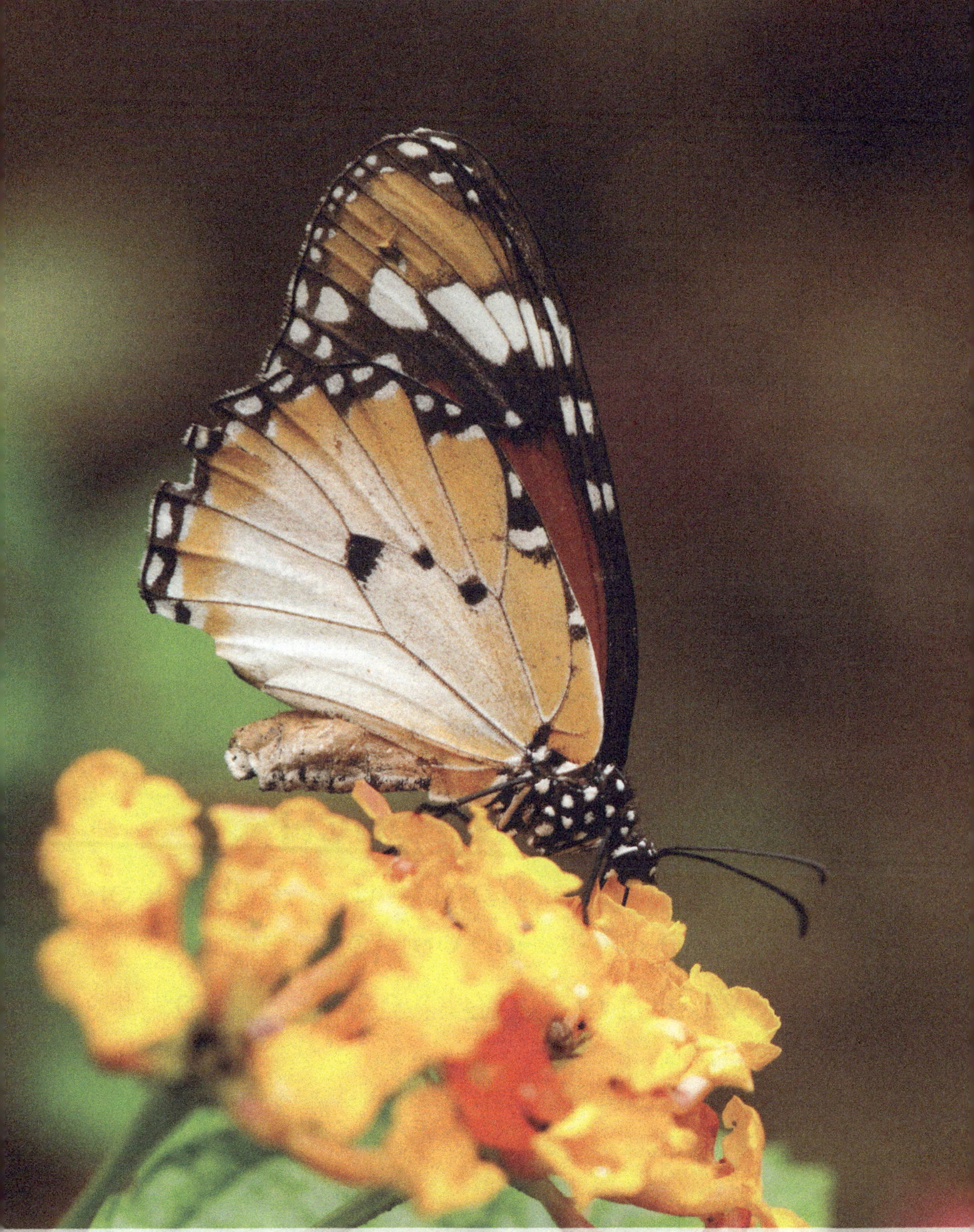

Fossils show this species is 2.5 million years old!

THANK YOU FOR READING!

WATCH THE ACCOMPANYING VIDEO

Scan with your phone's camera.

GRAB YOUR FREE BONUSES

Scan with your phone's camera.

STAY IN TOUCH

We'd love to hear from you - feedback or ideas? Reach out to us at:

skye@mail.silverdovebooks.com

SILVER DOVE
BOOKS

Made in the USA
Monee, IL
11 November 2026

68350826R00046